HER BLOOD IS GOLD

AWAKENING TO THE WISDOM
OF MENSTRUATION

HER BLOOD IS GOLD

AWAKENING TO THE WISDOM OF MENSTRUATION

LARA OWEN

FOREWORD BY

CHRISTIANE NORTHRUP, M.D.

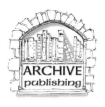

ARCHIVE
publishing

2008

This book was first published as
Her Blood Is Gold: Celebrating the Power of Menstruation
(HarperSanFrancisco 1993) and
Her Blood Is Gold: Reclaiming the Power of Menstruation
(Aquarian/Thorsons 1993).
A revised and expanded version was published as
Honoring Menstruation: A Time of Self-Renewal
(The Crossing Press 1998).

This edition by Archive Publishing
includes all of the second edition, with the addition of previously
deleted material from the first edition.

www.archivepublishing.co.uk

(Unit 3 Stone Lane Ind. Estate, Wimborne, Dorset, BH21 1HB)

Text © Lara Owen 2008
The rights of Lara Owen as author have been asserted in accordance
with the Copyright, Designs and Patents Act 1988.

A CIP Record for this book is available from
the British Cataloguing in Publication data office

ISBN 978-1-906289-07-2   Hardback
ISBN 978-1-906289-06-5   Paperback

To contact the author, please visit her website,
http:// laraowen.com

Printed and bound by Dardedze Holography

DEDICATION

This book is dedicated to those indigenous people of the world who have kept alive the ancient knowledge of the power of the menstrual cycle. I am very grateful for their persistence, tenacity and courage in maintaining these teachings.

A NOTE ON THE TITLE

The phrase, "Her blood is gold", comes from the creation myth of the Kogi Indians, the only known surviving and intact pre-Columbian society, who live in a secret part of the Sierra mountains of South America. The Kogi say that the world was created by the Great Mother during her period. "Her blood is gold, it remains in the earth, it is fertility."

The Kogi are a mysterious, mystical people who consider themselves to be the guardians of the planet, and constantly perform rituals for the balancing of the world from their mountain home in the Heart of the World. Their observations of the recent changes in the natural world around them trouble them deeply, and they warn that the planet faces imminent destruction due to environmental damage.

Many thanks to Alan Ereira for his book on the Kogi, *The Heart of the World*, and for the documentary of the same name, which happened to be on the television as I was writing the last sentence of this book, and from which I took the title.

TABLE OF CONTENTS

ACKNOWLEDGEMENTS

This book has been published in three different editions over a period of fifteen years. As a result, many people have helped to make this work manifest in each of its incarnations, and my heartfelt thanks go to them all.

For various contributions of support, advice, wisdom, and encouragement, my thanks go to David Brown, Howard Rheingold, Hazel van Wijnan, Karie Brown, Leba Wine, Charlotte Pauli, Sara Halprin, Nisha Zenoff, Arny and Amy Mindell, Max Shupbach, Rhea, Paul Giancarlo, Andrew Murray, Gemma Summers, Jackie Redner, Noelle Imparato, Alyson MacGregor, Debi West, Chris Knight, Joanne Leslie, Nalini Chilkov, Kathleen Pouls, and David Garbacz.

Thanks to Swiftdeer for giving me the initial teaching on the power of menstruation that sparked my research, and to the women and men of the Navajo nation who shared their knowledge of the Kinaalda ceremony with me. Thanks to Tsultrim Allione for introducing me to the wisdom of the dakinis. Thanks to my good friend and spiritual sister, Victoria Cresswell, for being such an inspiring and constant companion on the journey. Thanks to the women who allowed me to include their stories in the book: Wendy Alter, Hallie Iglehart Austen, and the late Tamara Slayton, much missed in the world of menstrual wisdom. Thanks to Dr. Christiane Northrup for writing the foreword and for her work in taking awareness of women's innate wisdom into the mainstream. Thanks to all the women who have communicated with me over the years about their menstrual experiences: they have heartened me and encouraged my work.

Marion Russell, Marian Young, Barbara Moulton, Liz Puttick, Elaine Gill, Jill Schettler and the staffs of HarperSanFrancisco, Aquarian/Thorson's and The Crossing Press all contributed to the publishing of the first two editions, and I thank all of them for their enthusiasm and expertise. Thanks to Ian Thorp at Archive Publishing for creating this beautiful third edition.

FOREWORD
BY CHRISTIANE NORTHRUP, MD

In medical school, I learned how to manipulate and "regulate" the natural female cycle with powerful synthetic hormones. I learned, albeit indirectly, that the menstrual cycle is inherently untrustworthy, and responsible for all kinds of female woes. I learned how to be prepared when women came in to be "cured" from the effects of this female adaptation. I learned every possible thing that could go wrong with this cycle, and a corresponding way to stop the symptoms, usually with drugs or surgery such as hysterectomy.

But I never learned in medical school or residency training what I really needed to know if I were ever going to help women truly heal their menstrual woes at the deepest level. What I needed to know is the subject of this extraordinary book, *Her Blood Is Gold*, which eloquently shows us why the monthly cycle of menstruation is a microcosm through which we can understand – physically, emotionally, spiritually – our connection with nature and with the process of creation itself. Nature did not make a mistake when it comes to menstruation. We forget that without the female menstrual cycle there would be no human life on Earth. When you stop fighting your period and stop considering it a nuisance and a pain, a whole new world opens up... and the pain begins to abate.

When we stop fighting our natural monthly cycles, we realize that our periods contain magic and mystery that plays out in an incredibly fine-tuned dance each month. Then we are ready to begin to heal ourselves and our female heritage at the deepest possible levels. We come to see that any imbalance in our cycles is signaling an imbalance in our lives. And we become grateful for the message of healing that our bodies – and nature – are sending us.

Through the work of courageous women like Lara Owen, who have dared to address the culturally taboo subject of menstruation so gracefully, I personally reclaimed the wisdom of my own cycle, and was able to recover from years of debilitating menstrual cramps as well as health-destroying ideas about the menstrual cycle. As I healed myself, I was able to pass this information on to my patients and as a result have seen hundreds of other women heal from a wide variety of menstrual problems, a process which starts with rethinking menstruaton. Together we are all breaking the chain of pain and silence about this vital cycle that has been handed down to women for generations.

The first step towards healing yourself is being open to the idea that menstruation is an inherently worthy process. From there you'll soon discover the magic in your own cyclic wisdom. Through the beautifully written *Her Blood Is Gold*, Lara Owen has provided women everywhere, and those who love them, with a gentle guide through the tender process of reclaiming menstrual wisdom and the power of this creative process. May the healing message in Lara's graceful prose reach women the world over with its message of hope, wholeness, and celebration.

Christiane Northrup, MD FACOG
author, *Women's Bodies, Women's Wisdom* (Bantam 1994)
website: drnorthrup.com

PREFACE TO THE 1998 EDITION

This book has been a work-in-progress for the last decade. My first writing on menstruation was published as an article in *Whole Earth Review* in 1991, and two years later a book entitled *Her Blood Is Gold* was published. Both of these works have been incorporated into the book you are reading now.

In the past few years there have been some gradual but perceptible changes in our collective attitude to menstruation, perhaps shown most obviously in television commercials and magazine advertising, which are less coy and more realistic and explicit in their portrayal of the menstruating woman.

People seem less affronted by the subject matter than they were when I began doing research. They are more willing to examine the possibility that in Western materialist culture our commonly held notions about the menstrual cycle have been infected by centuries of misogyny. The taboo about discussing menstruation still exists, but it appears to be gradually dissolving, along with other prejudices about the body and sexuality and gender.

I hope that these subtle changes in attitudes to menstruation presage a greater shift in how we collectively value, affirm, and accept female experience. The relationship between menstruation and power is still held very much under the surface of mainstream awareness, and most cultural references to menstruation continue to be couched in the terminology of pathology.

Reintegrating a truly feminist, woman-honoring perspective on menstruation means turning a whole system of thought upside down. It means saying that a cyclical change in feelings and body sensations is valuable and interesting; it means saying that the emotions women experience premenstrually carry useful information and should be paid attention to; it means acknowledging that a menstruating woman has access to sacred energy, and that if she wishes, she should have space and time to explore this dimension of experience.

The ramifications of such a shift would be truly radical. For many reasons, including ecological and cultural survival, I believe the system of thought which has caused women to adapt to a non-cyclical reality needs to be turned upside down, for the good of us all.

We menstruate more now than at any time in human history. Girls are starting to menstruate earlier due to protein-rich diets and hormones in food; women are less likely to die young; we have fewer children and therefore spend less time not menstruating. Increased work and family stresses, in addition to more periods, mean that women are more physically and psychologically vulnerable to negative attitudes to menstruation. So it is more important than ever that we investigate ways to make our periods physically, emotionally, and spiritually healthy.

Lack of recognition of menarche (the first period) is gradually being acknowledged as a source of self-esteem problems in adolescent girls. That the self-esteem of girls plummets at puberty has been well-documented in recent years, and is implicated as a cause of the terrifying epidemic of eating disorders among young women. There is also a link between school absenteeism and menstruation, strongest in the first year after menarche and caused as much by embarrassment, depression, and fear of blood showing on clothing as by any physiological symptomatology.[1]

In the majority of cases, menarche remains an unritualized, uncelebrated non-event, and as a society we have a long way to go toward making the first period a time which supports a young girl and ushers her successfully into her adolescent years and indeed, her womanhood.

Although it might seem a daunting task to remedy so many centuries of female belittlement and misunderstanding, there is much we can do. By drawing from pro-feminine traditions, and by creating rituals and behavioral changes appropriate to our time and culture, we can foster an atmosphere in which women feel empowered to respect, value, and enjoy the many gifts of the menstrual cycle. There is potentially an enormous ripple effect from such behavioral and attitudinal changes: by examining our prejudices and becoming more conscious about the ways our behavior perpetuates distrust and disdain for the natural processes of the female body, we can generate an increased respect for all matters feminine.

To that end, I have used the opportunity of enlarging my original work to add more information about concrete steps women can take to get into better relationship with their periods. This information is based on my own experiences and on the correspondence and teaching contact I have had with women all over the world. Some of these women had been quietly doing their own informal research and having their own experiences, and were very willing to share this information with me. Some of them had never thought about the matter consciously before reading my work, but once given the impetus were overjoyed to realize that there was more to being a woman than they had been taught. Over and over again I have been told, "I always had this feeling there was more going on with my period, and I just never heard anyone talk about it."

This book also includes a lengthy section on self-help for menstrual symptoms, and more detail in areas that I have studied further – chiefly cross-cultural perspectives and menarche rituals.

Studying menstruation is a reminder of the paradoxical human truth that just as we are tribal beings who all behave pretty much the same, so we are unique individuals with our own particular perceptions of reality. With that essential paradox in mind, this book comes with the following caveat: while certain aspects of my experiences with menstruation, and those of the other women included in this book, are universal, you will have your own unique reality and experience. The recommendations I make in this book are not rules; they are suggestions and guidelines based on many years of observation.

In this field, as in so much of life, we have to be careful about getting too rigid. While it is crucial for the well-being not only of women, but also of society, that we reincorporate ancient wisdom about the power of menstruation, we have to make it work for us in the present. This is a complex issue: for most of us, finding out what we genuinely want to do when we menstruate is very hard, because our thoughts are so overlaid with centuries of patriarchy and misogyny that have been integrated deeply into our collective psyche. For a woman to be spiritually awake, at home in her body, and psychically whole (a virgin in the true sense of the word: entire unto herself), she has to grow out of being primarily guided by principles of accommodation to others when these are not in her best interest.

The essential message of this book is this: if you take some time out to center yourself during your period, you will meet the genuine core of your being. From that authenticity you will naturally make choices in life that strengthen your spirit, heal your body, and honor the needs of your soul.

Lara Owen
Topanga Canyon,
November 1997

INTRODUCTION

The assumption that lies behind this book is that life is, on balance, a Good Thing, and that the processes of being female are likewise essentially a Good Thing. For the past few thousand years, certainly in Judeo-Christian culture (and in many others), being female has been seen as a Bad Thing. We have had a lineage of descent that honors the male over the female, and a preference for giving birth to sons. Consequently that which is special to the female has tended to be denigrated, whereas that which pertains to the male has been prized and respected.

Imagine how the world would be if men had periods and gave birth. The alchemy of producing blood every month would be recognized as a sign of the fertility that would be every man's pride and joy. Instead, what we have is a world in which menstruation is commonly referred to as "the curse" and where women do everything they can to disguise the fact that they are bleeding, often to the detriment of their health and well-being.

This book is the story of my journey into the menstrual mysteries, which I undertook unconsciously in the beginning, and later, as I began to realize what was happening to me, with more intent. It also includes the stories of several other women who, like me, tumbled down the rabbit-hole into the center of the earth, and found that their blood was a key into the heart of the Goddess.

Some years ago I began to understand the relationship between my thoughts and my physical health, and I realized that my sense of myself as a woman was warped and distressed by my thoughts, many of which were so automatic as to be unconscious. Even though I had been raised in a family that was relatively non-sexist, and had had many educational opportunities, I lived in a society that, even today, gives women the sometimes subtle, sometimes overt, message that they are inferior.

I began to have a fantasy of living at a time when there was not a thought in the collective that women were in any way lesser than men; a time when the processes of the female body were revered and respected. As I dreamed into this other reality, I realized that my whole body would be affected, and that not a cell in my being would have been formed out of ideas of female inferiority. This was a radical thought. Imagine not having a trace, a smidgen, hiding anywhere in your cells or your thoughts, that would ever imply that there was anything to be ashamed of about being female. That's what I want, I thought. I want to live like that. I want to really honor and discover the richness of my femininity, and I want to glory in it, revel in it. I want to dance with the mystery of my wondrous alchemical womb.

As a result of this journey – which I am still, of course, on – I now have a very different experience of being a woman, of menstruating, of the moon and the earth, of my body, my psyche, and my spirit. On the way I have learned how to get in touch with the wounded woman within, who bears the wounds that we all carry from growing up in a patriarchal culture. I have learned some ways to heal those wounds, and to begin to access the enormous strength that has been obscured by our ignorance of the power and beauty of the monthly cycle. I have learned that if I take time out for myself when I am bleeding I can access a centeredness and a wisdom within that feel eternal. Recognizing the value and pleasure of my periods has been a real opening for me into a deep appreciation of being a woman. The whole process has shifted from being something that I found mildly disgusting and certainly inconvenient, to being an natural time for assessment, clearing, and preparation. It has become a time when I process the last month and prepare for the one coming. I look forward to my period as a time when I am most likely to be able to seek creative solutions to difficulties in my life – provided I make the space for it. This process has been so transformative for me that I am excited by its potential for the healing of other women.

*   *   *   *

The book is divided into five parts. The first, Beliefs and Attitudes, begins with an exploration of our current perspective on menstruation in the Western industrialized world, seen from the personal angle of my own initiation (or rather lack of) into menstruation and fertility, and then from the collective angle of the development of patriarchal culture, the subsequent diminishment of female reality, and the role of industrialization in severing us from our cycles. Then I take a look at the eternal archetypes that underlie our conditioning, and are associated with menstruation throughout time and in cultures the world over, in particular the Moon and Blood, the Earth and Snakes. Chapter Three discusses the behavior and attitudes of societies that have a positive view of menstruation: cultures that see woman's monthly blood as a form of gold, a source of richness with the potential to nourish both physical and spiritual life.

Part Two, Reclaiming the Cycle, is about being a woman today and how our health and well-being are damaged by our attitude towards the menstrual cycle. I discuss ways to work creatively with menstrual symptoms so that we can heal ourselves and also discover what is useful behind our premenstrual rages and our cramps and lethargy. I look at what it is about our lifestyles that so readily creates menstrual disharmony, and how by reclaiming the natural impulses of the cycle we can gain not only physical health, but also psychological awareness and spiritual insight.

Part Three, Rituals and Recommendations, describes ways to peel away the surface layers of our conditioning and get down to our innate knowledge of the power and beauty of menstruation – knowledge that is in all of us, and which is an intrinsic part of having a positive experience of being a woman. Chapter Seven focuses on the practical steps involved in learning to menstruate with more consciousness, describing the four phases within the period itself, and dealing with issues like managing retreat time and using cloth menstrual pads. Chapter Eight goes deeper into a variety of ways to help us honor our bleeding and gain deeper awareness of our own individual experiences through keeping a journal, dreaming, rituals, meditations and working on creative projects. Chapter Nine is a concentrated compendium of natural remedies for menstrual symptoms and contains wisdom from many healing traditions.

In Part Four, Waking up to the Power, three women tell their stories of awakening to the mystery and magic and healing of menstruation. Wendy Alter was a chemical engineer with NASA who changed her lifestyle after recovering from breast cancer, and in the process discovered that her period was the strongest time for her to contact the depths of her nature: depths of feeling and insight that she had felt completely cut off from and that she recognized she had abandoned in her search for career success in a scientific world. Tamara Slayton, a pioneer in the field of menstrual education, taught women about the value of getting in touch with their cycles for many years, and was director of The Menstrual Health Foundation. Hallie Iglehart Austen, author of *Womanspirit* and *The Heart of the Goddess*, is a pioneer of women's spirituality who works with earth-centered ritual to promote personal and planetary healing. All three women spoke with me openly about their own relationship with their bleeding, and explained how, in different ways, making a strong connection with their cycle empowered and healed them.

Part Five, Living Your Power, looks at how the conscious experience of menstruation intersects with the outer world, and discusses ways in which we can change our lifestyles to incorporate more attention to our cycles, in the context of our relationships with men, women, children, and the workplace. The book ends with a vision of a world in which women are free to menstruate in the way they want and where the wisdom of women is once again seen as a valuable social and political resource.

PART ONE

BELIEFS
AND ATTITUDES

CHAPTER ONE

A Brief History of Bleeding : Menstruation in Western Culture

THE PERSONAL STORY

I used to think that my periods were a nuisance, a messy intrusion that increased laundry and caused a host of unpleasant symptoms including exhaustion and debilitating pain. It interfered with my sex life, with athletic activities, and with my energy level. It caused erratic mood swings, irritability, and destructive, unstoppable bitchiness. It cost money, in pads and tampons to mop up the blood, in ruined clothes, in time away from work. It was a mean and sneaky saboteur that would always come at the most inconvenient time.

Despite this catechism of woe I wasn't entirely against it. When my period came, there was always a part of me that was pleased. It meant I was healthy and fertile and that everything was working properly. There was a sense of pride about bleeding that I felt strongly with my first period, but, in the absence of any external support, the feeling of pleasure dwindled away.

Growing Up

I don't remember when I first heard about menstruation, how I first found out that one day I would bleed and it would be a good thing, not an accident. It was mysterious and I wanted it to happen. It meant I would be almost a grown-up, and another crucial step closer to making my own decisions and living my own life. I wanted very much to leave home and create a different atmosphere for myself, I didn't know what it would be, I just had a feeling of space and excitement. It was confusing though, because there was also something dark about beginning to bleed.

I remember my mother showing me the package of sanitary pads in the airing cupboard in the bathroom. They were for me, for when my bleeding started. There was a belt to hold the pad. I couldn't imagine having that pad between my skinny legs. But I didn't think about that. It was all too much for me. At school my friends started to bleed before me; all except my best friend, Nina. We were the late developers. Very smart, very cute, but no breasts, no blood, no boyfriends. My mother and her friends offered sympathetic comments: "Don't worry about it," they said. "They say that the later you start, the sooner you finish. You're lucky; it means you'll have fewer periods in the long run."

I didn't understand why that made me lucky. And why they thought that having periods was a bad thing. I hated their knowing looks, their world-weariness. What did they know? I wanted to grow up, and I wanted it now.

My First Period

My first period came in August, a month after my fourteenth birthday. I had a bath one evening and I looked down and there was a thin trickle of red on the inside of my thigh. I went downstairs. My mother was in the hall. Still on the stairs, holding the stair-rail, clutching the towel around me, feeling a hole where my stomach used to be, I said, "There's some blood on my leg."

My mother said, "It must be your period. Oh dear, I used those pads myself last month when I ran out." She held out her hands in excuse: "I'd kept them for so long."

It was a Sunday. The shops were closed. I don't remember what happened, we must have found a pad somewhere. My mother was kind to me, but somehow I felt like a nuisance. I felt empty. Then I felt very excited. I felt special. No one said very much. I carried on bleeding. I felt empty again.

When school started again I told my friend Nina. "I had my period," I said, trying to sound casual. She looked at me angrily: "I suppose you think that makes you something special." I stepped back, shocked. Well, yes, it did, but I didn't want to upset her. The little fragile balloon that was my pride in my womanhood deflated even more. I was just having a period. It was nothing special. Who did I think I was anyway? A friend of mine who is Jewish told me that when she had her first period her mother slapped her on the face. Reeling with shock, she said, "Why did you do that?" Her mother replied, "I don't know, it was done to me by my mother. It's tradition." Another friend said that she had been told by her grandmother that this traditional slapping was done so that the girl would always remember this important moment in her life. And yet another told me that it was so the girl would realize that she had now left childhood behind, and that adult life is hard and full of suffering.

To be hit on the face when first you become a woman – what an interesting statement about how womanliness is regarded. Perhaps it is intended to remove the feeling of pride that comes with the first blood.

Something else took away that feeling of pride for me, and I think it was the absence of ceremony. It felt to me, internally, that something truly amazing and magical was happening, and yet everyone around me treated it as a commonplace. I felt a sense of achievement, mingled with excitement, curiosity, and embarrassment; I also remember a vague awareness of a vast and gaping unknown future. Intuitively I knew it was a massive landmark in my life, and yet no one said anything about it, other than to give me some sanitary pads. I think my mother was pleased – after all, it meant I was healthy and growing up normally – but I needed more than that. I needed a ceremony, a party, some joyful public recognition of this huge event in my development. But nothing happened. As the months went by I felt more and more the shame and embarrassment, and less and less the excitement and the pride that had glimmered for a moment with the first blood.

Becoming a Woman

When I had my period I often felt fuzzy and found it hard to concentrate on my schoolwork. When I had important exams coming up my mother and I went to see the doctor and he gave me pills to stave off my period until after the exams. It worked a treat, and I passed all my exams. But my periods became strangely irregular, and I remember several months of very heavy bleeding every two weeks. I have a dim memory of lying in bed and feeling all this blood pouring out of me. Just as we were going to go back to the doctor, my periods calmed down, and I went back to being regular again. I don't think that either my mother or I ever considered that the pills I had taken might have upset my cycle. This was in the days when medicinal drugs were a completely Good Thing, when we were grateful of their miracles and ignorant of their insidious side-effects. Then I started to have really bad pains with my bleeding and so more drugs were prescribed for the pain, and not just painkillers but new hormonal drugs. I entered a vicious circle of using haphazard doses of hormones to control my already confused hormones which in turn led to more cramps and more bleeding.

"It'll settle down when you get older," said my mother and her friends, trying to console me, "When you get married, and have children." But marriage and children felt so far away when I was sixteen that this was little consolation.

It was miserable. Becoming a woman seemed to be an unmitigated drag. I wanted to travel; at sixteen Nina and I hitch-hiked round the south of England, and at seventeen we caught trains to Paris, to the south of France, to Italy. Everywhere we went we were harassed by men – on trains, on buses, on the street. It was awful. I hated it. It was totally impersonal and vaguely disgusting. I was still a virgin, and I felt confused and abused by the way men leered at us, tried to feel us up on the bus in Florence, and tried to persuade us to come back to their place instead of to the Youth Hostel.

I wanted to be a boy really badly. My friends who were boys could hitch-hike alone, could travel alone, without having to develop a steely look and fast reflexes like I did. When I was eighteen I went to live in Paris. After several months of navigating the Metro alone, I caught a glimpse of my pursed face in the window of the speeding train and realized that I was becoming ugly in my effort to keep all these men away from me. This was during the early seventies, in that brief moment during the era of free love just before the rise of feminism, when sexist behavior was still overt and widespread. I had been raised to be polite and I had no model of how to talk back to people who were intrusive and rude. I was vulnerable, and struggling to have my adventures in a male world.

So periods were just one more inconvenient part of being female. All I knew about menstruation was that it was a mark of being a woman and meant that I could (horror of horrors) get pregnant. At school, it was not a subject to be mentioned other than in the biology class. All the information I received was purely physical, apart from occasional crude jokes. You had a period because you weren't pregnant, and the menstrual flow was simply the discarded lining of the womb, provided for a possible fetus. My friends and I discussed it and, in the absence of further information, decided that the female body was poorly evolved, all that blood and fuss for years and years when you needed only to do it once or twice in order to have children.

And then there was that lurking uncomfortable shame that was somehow mixed up with the whole experience. At home, my periods were something to be kept secret from my father and brothers. If I had to mention it, I would use a hushed voice and preferably talk to my mother when we were alone. Shortly after my periods had begun, we were going on a family trip, and I had to ask my father to stop the car so that I could go to the pharmacy. Of course, he wanted to know what it was that I needed to buy. I remember this awful feeling as I told him I had to buy some sanitary pads. It was a peculiar mixture of shame, pride, and total embarrassment. He was very nice about it and, as far as I can remember, never said anything to make me feel that there was anything to be ashamed of, but somehow there was always this shame in the background of my thoughts, and it colored my whole relationship with the outside world.

The picture society gave me through advertising was a confusing one. Tampon ads showed lithe girls in bikinis running gleefully towards the ocean and girls in tight white jeans jumping onto horses. This didn't mesh very easily with my experience of lethargy and cramps. And I knew that no one in their right mind would trust a tampon so much that they would go out for the day in white jeans. Pah! It must have been men writing those ads.

Yet somehow I felt that I *should* be like the girls in the Tampax ads, and that the way my body and mind behaved was somehow wrong; that a normal girl wouldn't feel any different when she had her period. There's nothing she'd like more than to scramble onto a horse and gallop off for an adventure while that nice little tampon allowed her to forget that she was menstruating at all. The embarrassing reality was that I couldn't even get a tampon inside me. Not only was I not fitting the stereotype, I was also failing with the equipment. I felt decidedly inadequate until I eventually succeeded. Then the process of imagining I wasn't having a period at all began in earnest.

Tampons and the pill liberated me to a certain extent from the worst of menstruation. When I was eighteen I went on the pill and taking it meant that my periods were very light and completely predictable. If there was some reason why I didn't want to have my period I could mess about with my cycle by taking the pill straight through. My friends used to do this, and it was recommended for athletes and women whose career performance might be adversely affected by menstruating. I shudder now to think of the casual way we manipulated our bodies to fit our will.

Tampons meant that I never had to really look at my blood. I just stuffed the thing in, it took care of the mess, and then when I took it out I could sling it down the toilet without having to even look at it. My natural curiosity usually interfered with this procedure, but the possibility was there for pretty much ignoring that you were having a period at all. I could do anything with a tampon in: go swimming, wear a skimpy bikini or tight jeans. I was always sexually active. My period didn't slow me down – no sirree – I wasn't going to let something like that get in the way of my pleasure. The great thing about tampons was that they soaked up the blood that was coming out so that if you timed it right and whipped out the tampon immediately before intercourse, there was hardly any blood to be seen. Of course, being on the pill helped with that too, because there wasn't very much blood in the first place.

These attitudes – that periods were essentially a nuisance, and that they should be ignored as much as possible – pervaded my thinking about my body and my femaleness. Even when I became interested in holistic medicine it was a while before I began to change my behavior when I was menstruating. I understood that I was growing up into a world where, for the first time in modern history, women could take on men in the outside world and be liberated from the drudgery of the kitchen sink and childcare. I felt that I should make use of all the wonderful advances in medicine and hygiene that made it possible for me to pretend that, biologically, I wasn't really a woman after all. I owned my sexuality at last, but at what an enormous cost.

My journey out of this conditioning took over ten years, and I think it will probably be a lifetime task to work through and out of the myriad of insidious negative ideas about femaleness. At every new stage of my life I expect I will encounter denial and distrust in the essential nature of female experience. That is what living at this point in history is about, for me, and for many women.

THE COLLECTIVE STORY

So how has it happened that we think so little of the physiological processes of women's bodies? That we think that the best way to relate to monthly bleeding is to ignore it as much as possible, to walk around with cramping bellies and miserable minds, as though that were the lot of woman, and best to grin and bear it. This attitude is rooted in the denial of female reality that runs through the core of the history of the past few thousand years.

The world wasn't always dominated by patriarchal attitudes. Recent archeological findings tell us that there was a time when women and men worshipped the Great Goddess, the Earth Mother, and when images of the creative and fecund female were carved into stone and treasured.[1] As far as we can tell, about 5,000 years ago, militaristic groups from the Middle East began invading the peaceful, agrarian, Goddess-worshipping societies, beginning a long-term swing on the pendulum of human history. As the pendulum swung away from the Goddess and toward male-oriented values, it seems that the position of women in society became progressively worse, and aspects of life relating to the female were denigrated.

Over time this led to an association of shame with the body (always associated with the female, the Goddess, the Earth, feelings, and sensations) relative to the mind (associated with the male, the God, the sky, the world of ideas). Over the past few thousand years, all the mainstream religions in the world have become patriarchal (to varying degrees) and all of them value the intellect and the spirit over the body and the instincts. The old knowledge persists in the esoteric branches of the world religions, but the mainstream is primarily mind and sky oriented. God lives up there, not in the Earth. And there is pretty much a global consensus that He is Male.

Shame about the body, and shame about being female – it pretty quickly adds up to shame about menstruation. There is a shame that women carry simply for being women. The shame of women was bigger than the shame of men right from the first book of the Old Testament (a guidebook for life written by men and translated and interpreted by subsequent men). In fact, in the mythic version of history presented by the tale of Adam and Eve, male shame wouldn't even exist if it weren't for women. (And we do well to take these tales seriously, for although they may not have a basis in fact, they are the cornerstones of our belief systems.)

The book of Genesis tells us how the snake came to Eve and told her that the reason God had forbidden them to eat from the tree in the middle of the garden was not, as God has told them, because if they did they would die, but rather to prevent them becoming Gods themselves.

"Of course you will not die," said the serpent, "for God knows that, as soon as you eat it, your eyes will be opened and you will be like God himself, *knowing both good and evil*."

And Eve seeing that the fruit was *"desirable for the knowledge
it would give,"* picked some and ate it and then gave some to her
husband and he ate it too (Genesis 3: 4-6).

In the Middle Ages society became increasingly patriarchal. In
order to give religious support to the establishment of the
patriarchy there was some subtle – and some not-so-subtle – re-
creation of the old myths. Women were cast as the corrupters, the
Jezebels, to be feared and denied by the servants of a very male
God. The story of Adam and Eve was distorted so that knowledge
of good and evil was taken to mean knowledge of sex. Eve had,
through her wicked seductive powers, tricked innocent Adam
into falling from grace, and not because, as you remember, she
wanted knowledge. Oh no, it now became abundantly clear that
what Eve had been after was sex. The harlot! The problems of
humankind became, even more clearly, all Eve's fault. The curse
that God inflicts on Eve, "I will give you great labor in
childbearing; with labor you will bear children. You will desire
your husband, but he will be your master" (Genesis 3: 16), was
extended to include menstruation, which became the monthly
"curse" through which Eve paid for her sins.[2] I was educated in a
Church of England primary school in the 1960s, and I remember
being taught that Eve was the corrupter of Adam: she was the
temptress and the one who made the decision to eat the apple.
And although sex wasn't mentioned explicitly, all the pictures in
the books showed Adam and Eve naked, with Eve looking
seductive and sly while Adam was cast as a hapless man who was
putty in a woman's hands. That highly potent image was one of
the first images of woman that I was shown, and it was used to
illustrate the creation myth that lies at the basis of our cultural
identity. Small wonder that it has taken much unraveling to
discover the layer upon layer of distrust and ignorance of the
processes inherent in being a woman. We have had our own
bodily experiences so distorted that we have come to believe the
distortion rather than believe our own experiences.

The rise in power of the patriarchal religions did not happen
overnight. Pagan earth-centered religious practices, based on
ancient wisdom, continued to thrive, especially in Northern

Europe, well into the Middle Ages. Then Christianity became predominant, aided by social and economic changes and the terrors of long-term wars and the Black Death. The Inquisition brought about a period of unbelievable violence against heretics and thousands of so-called witches were killed with great brutality. With them died the visible remains of the Goddess religion and much of humankind's knowledge of midwifery, herbalism, agriculture, and spiritual practice based on natural laws.

After the takeover of European religious life by Christianity, the next major shift affecting the status of women was the Industrial Revolution. In nineteenth-century industrial Britain and North America, women were divided into two cultural stereotypes – the stoical breeder-worker, and the feeble little woman. One slaved away in the mills and factories, while the other languished on a sofa clutching a phial of smelling salts to her soft and tender bosom.

For the working woman, menstruation was a nuisance that cut down on her productivity. If she was earning wages by the hour or by the piece, then resting or relaxing in any way during her period was a luxury she could not afford. The poor have always had to work whether or not they have felt like it. However, in pre-industrial rural life, workload was related to seasonal flux. At harvest time everyone worked like the dickens; in midwinter there was virtual hibernation while the land lay under frost and snow. In a matter of decades, workers in Europe and America shifted from living in a culture which responded to the rhythm of the moon and the sun to one in which work was determined by the clock and by machines.

This had a particular effect on women, who had been used to greater autonomy in shaping their work day. If you are in charge of your own working environment – your home or small farm, for example – you can tailor your work to suit shifts in energy and disposition. This ability to adapt workload to one's inner rhythm disappeared with the industrial revolution, which tied workers to a concept of productivity based on the operation of machines. Unlike human beings, machines are not subject to seasonal and monthly fluctuations. The ideology of the industrial age adapted

human reality to that of machines, rather than making machines
fit the needs of humans.

For women who did not have to work outside the home, this
was not immediately felt, although it soon came home in the form
of exhausted husbands and sons. But the majority of working-
class women did have to go out to work, and for many of them
the demands of their jobs were extreme.

For middle-class women a very different concept of the female
arose. Perhaps in unconscious compensation for the sudden shift
into machine time, as well as because idleness still represented
status, nineteenth-century middle-class women were
characterized in medical and popular literature as feeble
creatures, prone to tuberculosis and neurasthenia. They were
believed to need protection from the outside world and from the
excessive stimulation that might be derived from reading novels
or riding horses. They were encouraged to rest during
menstruation. A medical book of the time advised: "We cannot
too emphatically urge the importance of regarding these monthly
returns as periods of ill-health, as days when the ordinary
occupations are to be suspended or modified." [3]

The correct behavior and treatment of middle-class women
during menstruation was the opposite of that considered
acceptable for working women, who were expected to carry on
working regardless of the time of the month. Class distinctions
were used by the medical profession to support this difference in
treatment. While middle- and upper-class women were seen as
sensitive and weak, working-class women were seen as
insensitive and tough, with a tendency to laziness that justified
their being whipped (sometimes literally) into productivity. This
phenomenon was most exaggerated in the southern United
States, with the vast difference in lifestyle between the black
slaves and the white wives and daughters of slave owners. It was
easier to have two medical models in this instance, for the
difference in race was used to support theories about the needs
and appropriate behavior of the two types.

Nineteenth-century medical concepts of the nature of the
female body and temperament laid much stress on the weakness

and volatility of emotion created by hormonal shifts. To the nineteenth-century physician, the womb and the ovaries were the most important organs in a woman's body. For example, Dr. Frederick Hollis wrote in 1849: "The Uterus, it must be remembered, is the controlling organ in the female body, being the most excitable of all, and so intimately connected with, by the ramifications of its numerous nerves, with every other part." [4]

Similarly, in 1870, Dr. W. W. Bliss waxed lyrical on the wonders of the ovaries: "Accepting then, these views of the gigantic power and influence of the ovaries over the whole animal economy of woman, that they are the most powerful agents in all the commotions of her system; that on them rest her intellectual standing in society, her physical perfection, and all that lends beauty to those fine and delicate contours which are constant objects of admiration, all that is great, noble and beautiful, all that is voluptuous, tender and endearing; that her fidelity, her devotedness, her perpetual vigilance, forecast, and all those qualities of mind and disposition which inspire respect and love and fit her as the safest counsellor and friend of man, spring from the ovaries." [5]

As more and more women have gone out to work and as our society has developed in terms of sexual equality, the stereotype of the frail and dependent middle-class woman has faded. It still exists, but as the butt of derision rather than as a sign of wealth and status. We place a far higher value on productivity than on leisure, and it is no longer satisfying or economic for most women to stay at home.

Modern feminism initially rejected ideas of hormonal influence on women. It is not surprising that feminists reacted against the idea that women are different during menstruation, as such ideas had played a large part in chaining middle-class Victorian women to their sofas. If women were deemed unreliable because of the changes in their hormones throughout the month, then this supposed unreliability was used as a reason to keep them from positions of power.

But our need to gain equality with men in the working world may have led us to throw some good ideas out with the bad.

There is usually at least a glimmer of truth in any ideology, and the physicians of the Victorian era were not completely wrong when they emphasized the importance of menstruation in women's overall health, the relationship between the womb and the psyche, and the wisdom of rest during the period. We have tended to reject all of this because it reminds us of the time when the lives of women were more controlled by men, and because it smacks of old arguments that kept women tied to the home and powerless in the outside world. We have also, quite rightly, rejected the idea that the natural processes of being female are a sickness. But to say that something is not a sickness is different from ignoring it altogether. By ignoring menstruation in reaction to the ideas of the Victorian era, perhaps we have lost touch entirely with a lingering thread of awareness of its value in women's lives.

The changes that have taken place in the lives of women over the past forty years may look like a revolution, but in many ways it has been an assimilation. Women seeking power in a male world have tended to do so by becoming pseudo-men. Perhaps unwittingly, feminism has played a part in the suppression of menstruation. Germaine Greer in "The Female Eunuch", her stirring tirade against the patriarchy, makes some important points about the taboos surrounding menstruation and how they reflect society's denigration of the female. But her conclusion is that menstruation is something that "we would rather do without" and that "no woman would menstruate if she did not have to". [6] This was very much the party line of feminism in the sixties and seventies and it was not until the rise of the women's spirituality movement in the 1980's that menstruation began to be seen as something sacred and meaningful.

In mainstream culture though, it is this idea of menstruation as inconvenience that has stuck, as women have increasingly adapted to work schedules formed by men and to a working atmosphere that developed within the context of a patriarchal society. When I discuss ancient ideas about the spiritual power of menstruation with successful and aspiring women, one of the biggest fears that I have come across is that this will in some way affect their myth of being "just as good as a man, and sometimes better". Many women don't want to go deeper into menstruation; they are scared of what they will discover. It suits them better to suppress their feelings with tranquilizers, to spray with vaginal deodorants to disguise the smell of blood, to numb their pain through painkillers, and to absorb their blood with tampons so they never have to actually see it. It's easier to be a successful woman in a man's world if you hardly recognize that you menstruate at all.

The technology of suppression – tampons, vaginal deodorants, sophisticated pain-killing and mood-altering drugs – has acted together with the myth of the superwoman to create a predominant cultural attitude that a menstruating woman is no different from one who is not bleeding. The trouble with all this is that it simply isn't true. Any woman remotely in touch with her body knows that when she is menstruating, and usually for a few days before, she feels different. And this is a fact of nature that ultimately cannot be denied.

CHAPTER TWO

Moon, Blood, Earth and Snake : Eternal Archetypes of Menstruation

Behind our culturally and historically determined attitudes and beliefs about menstruation lies an underlying web of symbols and myths that are a more permanent part of the matrix of human experience. The knowledge of these symbols lies deep within our bones, a legacy passed down in our genes from all the mothers who gave birth to us and our forbears, over millions of menstruating years.

No matter how we attempt to consign them to the shadow, the archetypes of the Moon, Blood, Earth, and Snake continue to pervade our unconscious life with their numinosity. They are all associated with the Goddess, and, like Her in Her most awesome and powerful expression, have held predominately negative connotations in recent history, particularly in the more patriarchal societies. These negative connotations are so powerful that it can be a stretch for us to even imagine that they are not fact, but are merely a view of reality, and not the only reality there is.

The Moon has been associated with lunacy and cyclical violence as much as with inspiration; its cycles have been seen to suggest inconsistency and unreliability rather than fluidity and the ability to experience a wide range of emotions.

Blood is seen as gore; people faint at the sight of it; we hide it on tampons and throw it down the toilet; we associate it with injury and death. Yet, in ancient times (and still in the Tantric tradition) menstrual blood was viewed as a sacrament symbolizing the wonder of life. As this is probably the most ancient of human sacraments: in all likelihood the origin of the Christian sacrament of the Blood of Christ lies in pre-Christian ritual involving menstrual blood.

The earth and nature have been seen as enemies, the earth as a resource to be exploited, and nature as a force to be tamed and governed. This collective failure to understand that the earth is a mother to be revered and respected has resulted in the current ecological disaster that threatens all life on the planet.

In Judeo-Christian tradition, the Snake has been assigned the most evil place of all the animal kingdom, as the cause of the fall from grace from the Garden of Eden. It once held power as the great symbol of death and rebirth, the magical one who brought knowledge of sexuality, of life and death, whose bite sent priestesses into visionary states and whose appearance presaged mystical and powerful events.

By exploring these symbols, their unconscious effects upon us, and their more ancient meanings, we can begin to peel off the layers of cultural conditioning that keep us from an intimate, positive relationship with femaleness. We can look at menstruation as if for the first time, with a spirit of inquiry and wonder. We can begin to experience the reverence that this magical flow of rich and fertile blood inspired in our ancestors. As Elinor Gadon tells us in *The Once & Future Goddess*:

> The word ritual comes from rtu, Sanskrit for menses. The earliest rituals were connected to the women's monthly bleeding. The blood from the womb that nourished the unborn child was believed to have mana, magical power. Women's periodic bleeding was a cosmic event, like the cycles of the moon and the waxing and waning of the tides. We have forgotten that women were the conduit to the sacred mystery of life and death.[1]

MOON

Before the advent of electric light, the full moon lighting up the night sky meant a time when one could walk easily at night, visit friends, hold social events, perform outdoor ceremonies, and observe wildlife for the hunt. The new moon, when the night is darkest, was a time of greater introversion, a time to go inside oneself; in many traditions, the new moon was a time of purification.

Many cultures have venerated the moon. Plutarch tells us that the priests of Ancient Egypt called the moon the Mother of the Universe, because the moon "having the light which makes moist and pregnant, is promotive of the generation of human beings and the fructification of plants." [2]

With the industrial age many associations with the moon died out of everyday life. But we only have to go back one or two hundred years to find evidence of the crucial relationship between the cycles of the moon and successful farming. In the British Isles it was believed that the wise farmer should "Kill fat swine for bacon about the full moon. Sheer sheep at the moon's increase: fell hand timber from the full to the change; horses and mares must be put together in the increase of the moon, for foals got in the wane are not accounted strong …fruit should be gathered, and cattle gelded, in the wane of the moon." [3]

Many cultures have understood the relationship of the cycles of the moon to the growth of plants, and this knowledge still survives. Biodynamic gardening, based on the teachings of Rudolph Steiner, is used by many gardeners in Europe as a guide to the relationship between horticulture and lunar phases, and in India it is still common practice in some areas to plant by the moon. [4]

The importance of the moon to the ancients lives on in a variety of traditions. The modern birthday cake comes to us from the Greek custom of honoring the monthly birthday of Artemis the Moon with lighted full-moon cakes. In Gaul, the crescent moon was an important symbol and the people made their communion cakes in a crescent shape. Modern France still makes them and calls them croissants (crescents), colloquially known as moon-teeth.[5] In pre-Islamic Arabia, the Moon Goddess was so important that her emblem came to represent the entire country and remains as the lunar crescent on Islamic flags. Today, the Arab equivalent of the Red Cross is called the Red Crescent.

The root word for both moon and mind was the Indo-

European word *manas, mana,* or *men,* said to mean mind, and an attribute of *Ma,* the primordial mother. Mana from heaven was divine food, spiritual blessing that flooded the body and nourished not only the soul, but also the physical being. Mana was also related to the Latin *mens,* meaning both mind and moon as well as a mysterious quality of spiritual power: nu-men. In Greek, *menos* meant both moon and power. *Men,* meaning month in Greek, is the root word for both measurement and menstruation.

The moon is associated with strong emotions: we talk of being moonstruck, of falling in love under the spell of the full moon. Many people are deeply affected by the full moon, and are more likely to have extreme moods, from elation to melancholy. The word *lunacy* derives from lunar, and many cultures believe that the moon itself creates madness in susceptible people, such is the strength of the emotion that it generates. The full moon triggers the werewolf's transformation, and the Moon card in the Tarot deck shows dogs howling under the moon.

In the traditional Tarot deck, the Moon is linked with danger and terror, whereas the Sun represents all that is good and bright and safe and strong. This is a good example of the shift in association we have had with the moon, and of the fear of night, darkness, and strong feelings that arises in a culture that fears the feminine. Once upon a time the moon was an inspiration, an aid to dreaming, and an evoker of rich emotion and poetic sensibility. Before we developed our fear of altered states of consciousness, *mania* meant ecstatic revelation, and *lunacy* meant possession by the spirit of the moon.[6] In patriarchal society, lunacy has become more associated with craziness and instability. The line between inspiration and mania can be a fine one, as we see in the lives of many gifted people, but the linking of genius and madness in Western society may actually arise as a result of the cultural tendency to repress particular kinds of emotional and creative energy. This repression can lead to neurosis and hysteria. The suppression of the wisdom of menstruation and of the moon may be the root of any lunacy that they bring.

The moon governs the night and therefore the darkness: that

which cannot readily be seen. The moon has a luminous beauty that pulls us into a different state of awareness. Whereas the sun lights the way for work and the round of daily life, the moon lights a different aspect of the human experience: the inner life, the imagination, the watery diffuse realms of the unconscious. This realm is of a very different nature than that of the sun. The Moon offers a more sensitive, delicate, fragile light: one that can distort as much as it can illumine, and its illumination is variable. At full moon the moonlight illumines everything; at new moon there is total darkness. This sensitive, fragile, variable feeling is familiar to women. For many of us it is typical of the premenstruum, when we are hypersensitive and volatile.

Our society worships the sun in that it favors the profligate use of energy, and behavior that is extrovert and outer-oriented. The quiet introvert, the poet, is not usually highly rewarded. Dreamers lose out in a culture which favors pragmatism and materialism. But as we can see from images in movies, love songs, and poetry, there is a nourishment at the soul level to be garnered from connecting with the moon. To sit under a full moon by the water and dream feeds the imagination, nurtures the spirit, and fills us with a sense of awe for life.

As Lindsay River and Sally Gillespie write, "while the Sun's light appears to have a constant and focused quality, the Moon's light appears *cyclic and diffuse* [italics mine]. There is a mystery in the Moon's soft-focused light which opens up the way to the magical illuminations of the unconscious. The wisdom attributed to the Moon throughout all cultures and ages is limitless". [7]

The associations that astrology holds with the moon are rooted in ancient ideas about the natural world. The moon relates to the feminine, the mind (especially the memory), emotional behavior, the home, the maternal, and the generative cycle.

In pre-patriarchal times many religions had female deities who in various ways represented and described the relationship of women to the moon, thus allowing women a sense of the divinity of their bodily processes. We are at a disadvantage today in that in most religions we no longer recognize, let alone worship, female deities. Women are therefore denied reassurance of the "rightness" of their cyclical, moon-related physiology. [8]

The ancient goddess Isis was always shown with the crescent moon. Diana/Artemis was the goddess of the moon, of hunting, of women and childbirth. She was an empowered woman and virgin in the sense of being owned by no man. She was a protector: of her human sisters, and of the animal kingdom.

The one female deity that is worshipped in the Western world, Mary the mother of Jesus, is traditionally depicted with a crescent moon at her feet, demonstrating the persistence of the symbolic relationship between the feminine and the moon.

The moon was considered the deity of women even as comparatively recently as the Renaissance, when it was said that women should pray to the moon, rather than to God, for what they wanted. [9]

In Scotland the full moon was considered the most fortunate time for women, and Scottish girls always got married at this time. They curtsied to the moon when they saw her, saying, "It is a fine moon God bless her." [10]

Many ancient cultures had a concept of the Triple Goddess: the Maiden, Bride, and Crone. The maiden is the virgin/young girl/princess, full of purity and promise, goddess of the new moon. During the waxing cycle of the moon she develops into the Woman, the fertile, creative, sexual, initiating priestess and queen of the full moon, who then, as the moon wanes, becomes the Crone, the goddess of death and of endings, of the period of moon-dark before the rebirth of the new moon. The ancients understood from this cycle that death always occurs before renewal and thus the Crone was seen as she who destroys in order to bring forth new life.

We can witness this cycle every month: the slim crescent of the new moon hangs delicately in the evening sky, and then she grows, like a pregnant belly, into the fullness of herself: an expression of abundance and fertility. Reaching a peak of roundness, lighting up the night sky almost eerily with her vibrant glow, the fullness completes itself and she begins to wane.

Slowly, slowly, she dwindles to nothing, and there is complete darkness in the sky. And then out of the empty darkness, the sliver of crystal clear new light can be seen, and she is reborn. This is a mirror of a literal process that takes place within the body and the psyche of every women every month, as well as for the living and dying process of which we are all a part.

The moon affects the flow of water by governing the tides. Our body fluids are also governed by the waxing and waning of the moon. The cycle itself is fluid; it is constantly changing. And this is what a woman's body is like: a continually shifting balance of hormones resulting in an ebb and flow of fluids: the blood that flows during menstruation; the dry phase after the end of the period; the runny egg-white mucus of ovulation; the juices of love-making; the tears of the premenstruum. Some women ejaculate a large quantity of fluid when they have an orgasm. This ebb and flow of fluids in the woman's body is a crucial part of her identity; it links her with the ocean and with the moon, with the waters of the planet, and with the cycle of the seasons.

Native Americans call menstruation the moon-time, and traditionally, menstruating women went to a moon-lodge to rest and meditate. In most cultures throughout the world the moon has been associated with women, most obviously because the average length of the menstrual cycle is 29.5 days, which is exactly the length of time that the moon takes to orbit the earth. The average length of pregnancy is 265.8 days, almost precisely nine lunar months. This falls fourteen days short of the forty weeks that today's doctors calculate as the length of pregnancy, but that forty weeks is measured from the beginning of the last period on the basis that theoretically at least, the woman could have conceived at any time after the onset of bleeding. In fact, she is most likely to conceive on the fourteenth day of her cycle making the actual period of pregnancy thirty-eight weeks, or 266 days.

The relationship between the full moon and ovulation was known in ancient cultures. Women of the Native American Yurok tribe of Northern California prayed to the full moon when they suffered from menstrual irregularity. It is probable that sitting out under the full moon triggered ovulation, and returned their cycles to normal.[11] In her book *Lunaception*, Louise Lacey describes how ovulation is triggered by exposure to light at night.

Ovulation is the signal for the release of the hormones that stimulate the build-up of the endometrium, the lining of the womb. The endometrium is shed fourteen days after ovulation; out of the whole menstrual cycle, this time period of bleeding fourteen days after ovulation is the most regular and widely experienced by women everywhere. This means that if the full moon triggers ovulation, then women will bleed fourteen days later, on the new moon. And indeed, it seems that this was generally the case in societies that did not use sources of light other than the sun and moon. When exposed only to natural light, women tend to menstruate with the new moon.

In societies with a female, earth-centered spirituality, such as that of the Native Americans, and ancient matrifocal Mediterranean cultures, the rhythm of the women's cycle was used as the basis for the ritual life of the culture. Rites of celebration and fertility were held during the full moon, when women were ovulating, and rites of seclusion and purification were held at the new moon, when women were menstruating.

These days we no longer live under natural light, and many factors conspire to shift our periods away from a regular cycle; however, it may well be that there have always been particular women, and also times in every woman's life, when menstruation occurs on the full moon. I have found that when my period coincides with the full moon it can be a very strong experience.

When I bleed with the full moon I am full of energy, full of juice, raring to go, happy, excited, full of sexuality and creativity. I am a channel for the bright light of the moon, and I sense her glow all around me. I usually require a time of peacefulness, but I need less time than when my period coincides with the new moon. My body wants to move, and I find myself dancing exuberantly.

When I bleed with the new moon I go very still and slow and retreat deep inside myself. It is more of a cleansing, a purification. I experience a drawing inside, a going deep within to the inner cave, the crucible of the psyche, a downward descent into the interior world, a time of the dark.

The elements of shifting energy, introversion and clearing out are always present for me when I am bleeding, but there is a different flavor depending on the moon's phase. I feel these differences most powerfully when my period coincides exactly with the new moon or full moon, and less so when it comes elsewhere in the moon's cycle.

Penelope Shuttle reported in her groundbreaking book, *The Wise Wound*, that she found her creativity to be particularly pronounced when she menstruated on the full moon. She and her co-author, Peter Redgrove, suggested that menstruation at the new moon is more connected to a biological creative cycle, and at the full moon more to an artistic creative cycle, or, at any rate, a creativity that is not oriented to the birth of a child, but rather to the birth of something else.[12]

These differences between full moon and new moon bleeding may partly explain why some women feel energized by their period, whereas others feel like withdrawing and being very quiet.

BLOOD

Like the moon, blood is one of the oldest and most central symbols for humankind, representing for us the magic of life. Blood is the primary symbol of the life force. It is found in the most ancient of art, as red ocher painted on figurines and on cave walls. Blood is one of the earliest sacraments used by humankind. In Paleolithic times, "The dead were buried in the fetal position with their arms across their chests, their bodies marked with red ochre, the pigmented earth, symbolic of life-giving blood". [13]

Blood has the power to create an impact. How does it feel when we see our blood coming out of our bodies? Blood is one of the manifestations of the mystery of our existence. Where did we come from? How did we get here? We know we are alive because our heart beats and pumps the blood through our veins. Our blood pulses and flows; blood moves through us continually.

We speak of drawing blood, of dripping blood, of people fainting when they see their blood. This occurs because of shock and of the fear of death overcoming us suddenly as we look at our blood flowing out of the body. Instinct tells us that when our blood is running freely from the body, we may die. The blood is supposed to be inside the body at all times, except for during menstruation and childbirth. The fact that women can bleed without dying added to their numinous power in ancient times.

We all have rich red blood throbbing through the veins, pulsating gently along the arteries and coursing through every cell. Carrying nutrients, dispersing waste, blood is the carrier, the conduit that enables our life force to flow.

Royalty was said to have purple or blue blood. Aristocratic blood, peasant blood, Irish blood, good blood – we still speak of lineage and ancestry in terms of blood. The concept of lineage is synonymous with the idea of shared blood. Tribal ceremonies often involve the mixing of blood to become symbolic relatives: blood brothers and sisters. At gypsy weddings in Europe the couple traditionally ate bread that held a drop of the other's blood on it, or even sometimes mingled blood directly from cuts on the hands or arms.[14]

The Moon and Blood are linked in astrological symbolism. Blood is shared by the family, and the family is represented astrologically by the Moon (genetic inheritance, the bloodline, is shown in particular by the south node of the Moon).

The color red has its own symbolism, which is related to ideas about blood. To the Chinese, red means wealth and is worn at weddings and other ceremonies where wealth is desired. The Maoris thought that anything became sacred once it was colored red, and Easter eggs were traditionally colored red. In Celtic Britain, to be stained red meant to be chosen by the Goddess as a king.[15]

In some cultures there is a belief in the mysterious healing nature of menstrual blood. Medieval physicians believed that the menstrual blood of a young girl could heal leprosy. They also thought that it acted as an aphrodisiac.[16]

Menstrual blood was considered sacred by many cultures. In the Tantric tradition men become spiritually powerful by ingesting menstrual blood. In the group rituals of the left-handed Tantric path, menstrual blood is taken along with red wine as a ritual drink.[17] The Taoists, Egyptians, Persians, and Celts all had similar beliefs.[18]

Menstrual blood has also been used as a fertilizer, and may have been a key in women's development of agriculture. In the autumn festival of the Themisphoria, the women of ancient Greece mixed menstrual blood with the seed corn. As Shuttle and Redgrove explain,

> "The women, who according to some sources invented agriculture, did so because only they had the secret of the strong fertility of the seed corn. The reason for this was that originally the women mixed the seed corn with menstrual blood, which was the best kind of fertilizer, before planting it. Since the men had no magic blood of this kind, they could not grow corn as well as the women could, any more than they could grow babies."[19]

In matrifocal cultures blood, was considered a carrier of magic because it represented the mystery of the life force. Elinor Gadon suggests that "the earliest rituals may have honored the menstrual cycle, the womb blood that nurtured the new life". [20]

Blood was the main symbol for the wellspring of existence and the mystery that sends us forth into this life. As such it was revered. The fact that women bled once a month meant that they were closer to this wellspring; this power innate in the female body was a large part of why the ineffable was revered in female form. Later, as cultures throughout the world became patriarchal, puberty rituals developed for males that also involved the shedding of blood, such as the subincision practiced by the aborigines of Australia and the breast piercing in the Sun Dance of the Lakota Sioux. These rituals may well have developed as imitations of the blood loss that women experience naturally.

In the Christian sacrament of communion, red wine symbolizes the blood of Christ. But red wine had been used as a symbol of the blood of the Great Mother, the Holy Woman, for centuries before Christ. In many cultures, ceremonies took place in which women and men would take the symbolic blood of life in the form of red wine, for example in the Dionysian mysteries and the Tantric rituals. Sometimes this was consciously acknowledged as being a symbol of the menstrual blood, the magical fluid out of which human life was created.

The custom of blood sacrifice is thought to have originated in the practice of using menstrual blood as a sacrament. As male priests gained power and the feminine perspective waned, so the power of menstruation, an exclusively female act, was set apart from the rituals of worship and reverence. Religion turned to the idea of an external force that needed to be placated by the offering of the blood of an animal or young person. This can be seen as a distortion of the more ancient knowledge of blood as representing the sacred nature of life itself. Offering the menstrual blood is entirely different from offering the blood of a being who has to die in order for its blood to be offered. Offering menstrual blood was and is an affirmation of life, a recognition of its sanctity, of its magic.[21]

It is possible that male envy of the blood released by women fueled many of the negative taboos around menstruation. The concept that menstrual blood is a pollutant is a distortion of the ancient idea that it was a sacrament.

EARTH

Whatever symbolism operates in the collective about the Earth tells us a good deal about the way women and menstruation are seen. In the vast majority of traditions, the earth has been associated with the feminine, and in ancient times and in pro-feminine cultures, was and is considered both female and sacred. Sometimes the earth was considered to have been created by a female being, a cosmic mother figure. The Kogi people of Columbia believe that the earth was formed by the Great Mother during her period, and that her blood flowed into the earth and became the precious gold in the seams of the Earth's rocky interior.[22]

The Earth Mother was recognized as the source of nutrition, of shelter, and clothing. Many cultures have shared a sense of the Earth as Divine Parent, whose gifts extend beyond the provision of physical nurturance and include moral and spiritual guidance. In Russia, instead of touching a Bible when taking an oath, a peasant would place a clod of earth on his head, invoking the curse of the Mother if he broke his word.[23]

In the Native American vision quest, the behavior of the natural world around one is seen as a source of special information. In that tradition, God – referred to as the Great Spirit – is experienced as being in the Earth, borne on the winds, and seen through the behavior of animals and birds, rather than as the Big Man up in the sky of the patriarchal religions.

The Earth, like the menstruating woman, has lost her status as sacred mother as humans have become increasingly "civilized" and distanced from nature. We have in many ways lost our instinctual relationship with the ground beneath our feet and as a result we are filled with fear of poverty and scarcity. Our over-anxious hustle for ever greater material wealth may in part result from this loss of connection with the source of our physical nourishment and well-being.

The Earth as archetypal mother, as symbol of Home, has been reconfigured and enlivened in recent years by, paradoxically and perfectly, the very technology that threatens the Earth's well-being. Photographs taken from outer space have given us a renewed sense of awe, and many astronauts have spoken of the immense beauty of this planet when seen from far, far away. It seems that in order to reconnect at a deeper level with our abilities to steward and respect our planetary home, we have to gain an extreme perspective, visually and viscerally, and go as far as to risk losing the very nurturing powers of the earth that we depend upon for our survival. It is these photographs of the earth taken from outer space which currently reflect back to us our collective image of the Earth as mother and as home.

As described above, the women of ancient Greece, and doubtless many other cultures, used their menstrual blood to fertilize the fields, and had an intense and intimate relationship with the land because they bled onto it. As women, we are of the earth in a powerful way. She and we are the nurturers, the givers of life. The Earth is our home, just as we have homes within us.

Within each woman there is a womb, which is a home for a new being, and when that womb bleeds, our connection with the earth is activated in a cellular and magical way. We have an instinctive relationship of similarity with her, and giving our blood back onto the earth strengthens this relationship.

When women share their menstrual blood with the earth, either individually or in ceremony, an enormous positive collective power is unleashed that can rebalance and heal the planet. When women bleed and put their blood on the earth, they act as a conduit between the generative forces of the moon and the receptive fertile energies of the Earth. Women link these two celestial bodies – the Earth and the Moon – through their lunar-related and earth-nurturing menstrual flow.

SNAKE

The snake, who renews itself by shedding its skin and who gets about by slithering along the ground, is a symbol of the energy of change and of the energy of the earth, and as such is both scary and inspiring.

It was a snake that persuaded Eve to eat from the Tree of the Knowledge of Good and Evil. For that crime, God banished the serpent, committing it to an eternal future of crawling on its belly in the dust. The Christian God of Genesis also changed the relationship between the Snake and Woman, "I shall put enmity between you and the woman, between your brood and hers". (Genesis 3:15) From the story of the serpent in the Garden of Eden onward, we have been conditioned to be repulsed by snakes.

In contrast, many of the earth-centered cultures of the world have had a reverence for the snake. They have seen within its cyclical shedding of the skin a metaphor for the birth/life/death cycle of humankind. The symbolism of the snake has also been used to illustrate the little deaths that we undergo during our lives – the shedding of childhood at puberty, the shedding of fertility at menopause, the shedding of relationships with the death of loved ones. That the snake lives on in a new and purified form after the skin has been shed has been universally used as a metaphor for the cleansing power of change and transformation, and also as a symbol of everlasting life.

The snake is therefore a symbol of the personal power that accrues from willingly going through the transformative fires of life, and agreeing to be transformed by the experience of living, rather than trying to hang onto the known. This personal power is anathema to patriarchal cultural structures, which work by diminishing the personal power of the individual, except for the few who rule from the top of the hierarchical pyramid.

In matrifocal societies the snake was a friend, ally, and helper of the Goddess, and of her priestesses and priests. In Ancient Egypt the hieroglyph for snake also meant Goddess. Priestesses used snake venom to induce trance, and would often have a snake familiar who lived with them, coiled in trance itself much of the time.

Women and snakes share a pattern of cyclical shedding. For the snake it is a skin that is shed, for the woman the lining of the womb when she menstruates. The skin is shed; the death of the potential babe gives rise to the rebirth of the woman.

The snake as a universal symbol of renewal gives us a vital clue into the menstrual mysteries. Our monthly shedding is a key to our own renewal, our health, and our personal power. Every month we have the opportunity to renew and refresh our whole beings, physically, psychologically, and spiritually.

CHAPTER THREE

Sacred Power :
Beliefs of Menstrual-Positive Cultures

In my twenties I trained to be a doctor of Chinese medicine. The discovery that the Chinese have a very different attitude to menstruation stimulated me to rethink my beliefs and practices. I learned that traditionally the Chinese recommend resting during menstruation, and that they consider the cause of many gynecological complaints to be faulty behavior during menstruation, for example getting cold, lifting heavy objects, overworking, and eating inappropriate food.

Until this point I hadn't really thought about my period very much other than to consider it a nuisance. Like everyone else I knew, I had been raised to grin and bear it and carry on as normal and to suppress my desire to lie around in a dream for a couple of days a month. I also suffered from bad cramps which I would usually treat with painkillers, although I knew that rest and a hot water bottle would soothe them; it was just that I couldn't allow myself to rest.

My Chinese teachers encouraged me to honor my body feelings, because they had a medical model that supported the idea of rest during menses. It was wonderful to discover a whole body of medical knowledge and folklore that recommended that I do exactly what I felt like doing when I had my period. I found that it was okay to indulge myself and to spend the first day or so of my period lying down and spacing out in a comfortable and quiet environment, sipping hot herb tea and allowing my body to have a rest. As I experienced the healing that began to take place in my whole body, I realized that the menstrual period is a natural time for women to rest, a time in every month when the body requests a time, a few hours at least, of relaxation. By cutting through this natural tendency and attempting to fit into a male-dominated work schedule, I had begun to make myself sick. Beginning to follow my body rather than ordering it around after me was a major shift. But that wasn't all; the discovery that not everyone thought the same way about menstruation opened up my own thinking. I began to realize that there was a wisdom inherent in the body itself, and that my own culture didn't necessarily have a very wise or useful attitude to the processes of being female. The recognition that my attitude to menstruation had developed in the context of a society that has diminished the female for several thousand years was a major step in the development of my understanding.

I realized that not everybody everywhere thinks that menstruation is an inconvenient event to be ignored, and not everyone everywhere thinks that it is yet more proof that women are inferior to men.

However, the Chinese model only went so far. It never approached issues of power and spirituality, and although the emphasis on rest was very useful, it kept me locked in a mindset that menstruation was weakness rather than strength. It was when I came across the teachings of the Native American tradition a few years later that I began to understand that something very profound was going on while I was lying about and spacing out; it wasn't simply that I was resting a tired body and rebuilding lost red blood cells.

THE NATIVE AMERICAN TRADITION

In the Native American tradition a woman is considered to be at her most powerful, psychically and spiritually, when she is menstruating. Resting during menstruation is seen in the context of one's attention being elsewhere. Your energy is focused on the spiritual plane, on gathering wisdom.

The different feelings that women have when they menstruate are understood to be part of something very meaningful about the cycles of the woman's body. In many Native American societies, before their traditional practices were suppressed, the women would often go to a menstrual hut (a moon-lodge) to pass the time of their bleeding.

Most of the women would bleed at the same time, usually coinciding with the new moon. In *Daughters of Copper Woman*, Anne Cameron describes the lives of women of the Nootka people of the Pacific North-West, and reports that the atmosphere in the moon-lodge was one of a holiday or party. The women would play games, and talk, and rub each other's backs to ease cramps. They would sit on special moss padding and give their blood back to the Earth Mother.[1]

It wasn't only a time for rest and relaxation, but also a time for gathering spiritual wisdom. In the tale of Tem Eyos Ki, a woman living at the time when the men of the tribe began to assume dominance over the women, it is during her seclusion during menstruation that she comes to an awakening. As a result of the wisdom she finds in the moon-lodge (called the waiting house by the Nootka), she emerges after four days and sings a song of great beauty and love that awakens the tribe to the imbalance between the men and the women.[2] This story echoes the Cherokee belief that the menstruating woman is performing a function of cleansing and of gathering wisdom, that is beneficial not only for the woman herself but also for the whole tribe.

One of the most inspiring accounts of menstrual beliefs and practices that I have read comes from a woman of the Yurok people of Northern California, paraphrased by Thomas Buckley:

A menstruating woman should isolate herself because this is the time when she is at the height of her powers. Thus the time should not be wasted in mundane tasks and social distractions, nor should one's concentration be broken by contact with the opposite sex. Rather, all of one's energies should be applied in concentrated meditation "to find out the purpose of your life" and towards the "accumulation" of spiritual energy. The menstrual shelter, or room, is "like the men's sweathouse", a place where you "go into yourself and make yourself stronger". The blood that flows serves to "purify" the woman, preparing her for spiritual accomplishment. A woman must use a scratching implement, instead of scratching absent-mindedly with her fingers, as an aid in focusing her full attention on her body by making even the most natural and spontaneous actions fully conscious and intentional: "You should feel all of your body exactly as it is, and pay attention." [3]

It was usual for most Native American groups to hold puberty rituals for the young women, and for many, these were the most elaborate and beloved of all their ceremonies. The puberty rituals of the Nootka graphically demonstrate the respect and reverence that they had for women. After a girl had her first moon-time there would be a big party for her. Then she would undergo a ritual of endurance, in which she would be taken far out to sea and left to make her own way home by swimming back to land. On arriving back at the shore she would be greeted by the whole village, and from that moment on she would be recognized as a woman, and seen as ready for the responsibilities of marriage and children. [4] The training for the physical aspect of the ritual was considered very important, as the new woman should demonstrate her capacity for patience and perseverance. [5]

The Navajo people still practice their puberty ritual for girls. It is called the Kinaalda, and is considered by them to be the most important of all their rituals. In the month after a girl has her first period, her entire extended family gather together for a ceremony that takes about four days. When I visited the Navajo nation in 1995, the women I spoke with estimated that perhaps half of the girls still have the Kinaalda ceremony, and they expressed their concern that it was not happening enough because of increasing pressures from mainstream society, and the logistical difficulties of getting the whole family together for several days at one time. A matrilineal culture, the Navajo consider the Kinaalda to be so important because when a girl becomes fertile, she brings new life to the people.

Every morning of the ritual, the girl gets up at dawn and runs toward the rising sun. Each day she is expected to run further and faster. During the days, an older female relative, in the role of "Ideal Woman", teaches her about the Beauty way, and molds her body through massage so that she will have a good figure. The girl is instructed in tribal wisdom about relationships between men and women, and about how to make a good wife.

The girl and her family – the men and the women – together prepare an enormous corn cake which they cook in an oven dug inside the earth, specially for the occasion. During the days of the ritual the girl is expected to take on a new level of responsibility for herself and for others.

On the last night, the shaman of the tribe (also known as the medicine man), comes to join the family, and everyone stays up all night praying for the girl, and for her family, and for the whole tribe. This night is considered very important for the well-being of all the people.

On the last day, the girl, who is seen as an emanation of Changing Woman throughout the Kinaalda, wears a traditional buckskin dress. Her hair is braided in a special way. Her first action as a woman is to hand out pieces of the hot corn cake to all the participants in her coming-of-age ceremony.

The rites of passage of the Nootka and the Navajo emphasize both physical strength and the development of character. This teaching seems so apt, and so lacking in our modern world. Our initiation of girls into womanhood is superficial in comparision: how to put on makeup, buying your first bra, using a tampon for the first time. Many women get married and get pregnant without having any sense of their own capacity for endurance, physically or psychologically. Small wonder then that so many girl-women elect to give birth with the aid of painkillers and a technology that robs them of the experience of their own strength. This lack of challenge and strengthening at puberty may also contribute to the self-hate that afflicts so many young women and leads to eating disorders, addictions, and depression.

THE PYGMIES OF THE CONGO

The puberty rituals of the Pygmies of the Congo, described by Colin Turnbull in *The Forest People*, also depict a culture with a positive view of women and of their power. Unlike the Pygmies, the nearby African villagers view the arrival of a girl's first menstrual blood as an evil omen, and "something best concealed and not talked about in public. The girl is an object of suspicion, scorn, repulsion, and anger". In contrast, the Pygmies greet menstrual blood as a symbol of life, and when a Pygmy girl has her first blood it is considered a gift. The whole group joins in a puberty festival called the *elima*, and as Turnbull notes, "the *elima* is one of the happiest, most joyful occasions in their lives". [6]

The *elima* involves all kinds of physical activities and much playing and running in the forest, as well as training by the older women in the elima house. The girls learn the songs of the women and they sing loudly through the forest, "so that everyone should know that they were the *Bamelina*, the people of the *elima*, girls who had been blessed with the blood and were now women". [7]

THE DAGARA OF BURKINA FASO

Sobonfu Somé comes from the West African Dagara tribe, from the village of Dano in Burkina Faso. She and her husband, Malidoma Somé, now live in the United States where they teach the knowledge of their people, especially concerning the importance of initiation at puberty, and about making good and deep relationships between men and women.

Among the Dagara, the initiation of girls is performed once a year for all the girls who have begun to menstruate in the preceding year, sometime between December and February. "During initiation you learn about many things; sex and intimacy are just part of this. Even after initiation, there is a long period of mentoring." [8]

The Dagara believe that the menstruating woman "carries

healing energy within her and has a tremendous ability to heal and see into things. In my village, people will seek help from such a woman. They will treat her with great respect". When Sobonfu was taught this by the elder women in her tribe, she says, "This discussion opened something infinite in me". [9]

The understanding of the value of menstruation extends to women supporting each other, by doing rituals for an individual who is having her period. "There is also the need for someone to contain the space for the mooning woman, as she could be channeling energies from different sources. Rituals take whatever form the woman having her period chooses. Some women will say: 'I want to be carried to this place in the village and have people sing and dance and rock me.' It's not something that is restricted. Both men and women can be involved in these rituals. She can ask them to do whatever she wants." [10]

THE BENIGN WORLDVIEW & ATTITUDES TO MENSTRUATION

Colin Turnbull notes that the Pygmies, unlike their village-dwelling neighbors, have "complete faith ... in the goodness of their forest world". "All that is needful is to awaken the forest (*through song*) and everything will come right." [11]

The Pygmies have a benign worldview; that is, they think of the forest in which they live as a place that will readily meet their needs for food and shelter, and also their needs for spiritual protection. They are completely at home in the forest, and they have a relationship of love and respect with their environment. This seems to be intricately related to their positive attitude to the feminine.

The Yurok and the Nootka also had a good relationship with their environment. They were well adapted to it, and the ocean and rivers and forests nearby gave them ample food. The Navajo today are committed to living in harmony with the land. Like the Pygmies, they see menstruation as a time of power, and the puberty of girls a time of strength and celebration.

It seems that a benign worldview is a prerequisite for a

positive attitude toward one's own world – one's own body – and most specifically, toward the female body, as that is a microcosm of the larger female body, the earth.

This is clearly reflected in the attitudes of these cultures to menstruation. It is interesting to note that as Western culture becomes more earth-conscious and awakened to the ecological damage that our lack of respect for the Earth is creating, the female is also becoming more respected.

Many indigenous cultures are aware of the threat to the earth's well-being posed by the modern era. The Kogi Indians of Colombia, who live in a secret part of the Sierra mountains of South America, have a complex, mystical worldview and a sense of guardianship for the planet. Like the other tribes mentioned in this chapter, they have a deep belief in the sanctity of menstruation, and go so far as to consider the blood of women equivalent to gold. The Kogi's message about the potential imminence of our mass destruction due to environmental damage is a stark reminder of how respect for the value of menstruation is directly related to the survival of life on this planet.

Menstrual beliefs and rituals have fascinated anthropologists for years, and there is a growing body of research on the subject. To find out more about different cultures and their perspectives on menstruation, read *Blood Magic,* edited by Thomas Buckley and Alma Gottlieb. There are also several other books mentioned in the bibliography at the back of this book.

PART TWO

RECLAIMING
THE CYCLE

Chapter Four

Healing the Wounded Woman

When I was growing up I swore that I would not turn out like my female forebears. My mother and grandmothers seemed to have a much more restricted life than the men of the family, and I could see that they commanded less respect as soon as the conversation veered from the personal to the world of ideas and opinions. I was a well-read, opinionated girl who placed a high value on intellectual respect, and I didn't see any reason why my opinion should have less weight than a man's. My parents supported me in this; they wanted me to have a good education and to have confidence in myself. I was smart, and I knew it.

In the outside world it was clear that it was the fathers who had the money and the power and the freedom and the control. I never saw any women who had a level of autonomy and control to match that of the men. The only women I knew who worked were the teachers at school. All other women were mothers. I promised myself that I would not have a life like that, where I had to subordinate myself to a husband and family.

The problem with breaking tradition in this way, albeit aided and abetted by my family, was that I tended to see everything about my mother's and grandmothers' priorities, skills, and worldview as somehow old hat, backward-looking, and emotional rather than intellectual. In rebelling against the image of womanhood as the supporter of men and the nurturer of the family, I threw out much of the value of the feminine. It took a conscious wish and deep inner work to begin loving myself as a woman and to stop running away from my female nature.

At school and university I was trained in an analytical model of perception which I valued above feelings and intuition. Growing up in the sixties and seventies meant that I was part of a generation that used experimentation with drugs to help shift our consciousness into an awareness of the value of the nonrational. This had the effect of somewhat compensating for the onesidedness of my education. But despite my explorations of different states of consciousness, as a teenager I had already made certain decisions about myself and my life based on an abhorrence of the female and the diminished role she was forced to carry in the society in which I was raised.

These decisions carried on into my twenties, often translated into an unconscious awkwardness with the female aspect of myself. I had no role models of the kind of woman I wanted to be. I was making it up as I went along, and sometimes the only way I could do what I wanted to do appeared to be by dispensing with the female within altogether. And in a subtle way, that translated into my sense of my body. I wore jeans most of the time, and I eschewed much of what would be considered female. I kept my home in good shape and I was sympathetic with my friends, but I valued my work in the outside world more than anything else, because that appeared to be what society placed most value upon.

By the time I was twenty I had been taking the the pill for about two years. I noticed that I was getting increasingly emotional and upset during my so-called period and these temporary bursts of hysteria felt very strange, as if I really wasn't myself. I decided to stop taking the pill and see if that had anything to do with it. I was also beginning to have fantasies about getting pregnant although that was, to my conscious mind, an impossibility. I was much too young, unmarried and aware that my friends who had kids young seemed to have a very difficult time. No, that was a Bad Idea, only entered into by irresponsible women who didn't know what to do with their lives and who resorted to their biological functions for something to do. Well, I was going to have a career and be a useful member of society, not a mere breeder.

The split in me between the instincts of my inner woman and my masculine-oriented social conditioning was severe. And I didn't realize it: I thought I was a feminist. It didn't occur to me, at that age, that the reason my less-organized friends with babies had such a hard time was because society was arranged in such a way that young women had very little power. And no-one seemed to be very interested in helping them. I really did think, and it is very painful to admit this, that it was their fault, that they had been stupid to get pregnant. I was going to be very careful that it didn't happen to me.

That was one part of me; the other side was flirting with the idea of pregnancy. So I came off the pill, partly because I suspected that it was messing me up and also because there was the glimmer of a reproductive drive stirring in my being.

After a couple of months I felt like myself again, and I realized that despite the convenience of the pill, I had actually felt cheated because my periods were so light. This was when I first began to realize that menstruating was an important part of my life, a rhythm that I depended on for my psychic and physical health, and that I ignored or suppressed it at my peril.

I became interested in the whole cycle, and investigated natural birth control. My bedroom was plastered with charts as I attempted to track my vaginal mucus flow. I never was very good about taking my temperature and I've always disliked thermometers. But I did begin to realize that if I took the time to tune in, I actually had a lot of awareness about what was happening in my body. I could feel a twinge over my ovary when I ovulated. I could track the subtle shifts in my sexuality, the levels of introversion and extroversion throughout the month. I began to understand that it was possible to befriend this mysterious cycle that had always seemed a burden to me. I liked knowing what my body was up to.

Despite the glimmers of awareness that this awakening brought, when I became pregnant a few years later I still had an attitude of neglect towards my body when its needs interfered with my work. I remember being extremely hungry but putting other things before eating. I miscarried, and the grief that I felt in my body for the lost baby and the frustration of a pregnancy cut short awakened me to my body and its essential femaleness in a shocking way.

This was an experience that set me apart from the world of men, and the intellect, in a stark and thorough way. I had no conscious resources within me to deal with the feelings that overwhelmed me. I was full of loss for a being that had at most been six weeks old. It didn't make any sense. But I could feel my body grieving in a powerful way. I cried endlessly, and was depressed throughout the rest of what would have been the pregnancy. All I wanted was to get pregnant again, but I didn't conceive. My husband didn't understand my pain, and I didn't understand or accept it enough to be able to explain it to him. I was lost in an unexpected sea of hormonal anguish. Being a woman was taking me into regions of feeling that were vast and uncontrollable. Why had no one prepared me for this? Why didn't anyone talk about the fact that a woman's physiology had such a powerful effect on her mental and emotional state? Was I some kind of aberration, or was this another of the facets of female experience consigned to the secret compartment of life?

One day an acupuncture client of mine said, "I had three mis-carriages you know, and every time I felt the most terrible grief. No one who hasn't been through it understands the pain of it."

I felt a bit better after that, and I realized that I didn't have a single woman in my family or circle of friends who had had a miscarriage and who could have reassured me from her own experience. But many of them had been through pregnancy and childbirth; if miscarriage could provoke such a flood of feeling, what on earth was giving birth like? I began talking to women and reading on the subject, and I began to see that while there was still a folkloric tradition that accepted the reality of mood swings and hyper-emotionality, this understanding didn't fit into the modern world. It seemed to be being taken less and less into account. Were women becoming less emotional, or was it that society refused to acknowledge the relationship between cycles and mood? It seemed to me that much of the richness of female experience was being cauterized by the machine age, by the linear mind that works in weeks rather than moon cycles, and talks of pregnancy as forty weeks rather than nine moons; by a society that calls a woman's blood-time her "period" rather than any of the more beautiful names that have been used in other times and cultures, the most often heard being *moon-time*, the term used by the Native Americans.

After the miscarriage my moon-time became extremely painful, both physically and emotionally. I had truly terrible cramps, and atrocious pre-menstrual rages. My marriage was falling apart, and the chief reason seemed to be our inability to understand each other's maleness and femaleness. We used to joke about men and women needing to live apart for their own sanity. But really, we each didn't understand or respect the needs and rhythms of our own gender. I would become enraged every month in order to send my husband away, instead of being able to say gracefully, "I would like some time alone when I am bleeding".

In my late twenties I discovered that I had cervical dysplasia (abnormal cells on the surface of the cervix), and the gynecologist wanted to cauterize my cervix. I was horror-struck, and my body recoiled from such a brutal procedure. Instinctively I knew that it would not going to be a healing for me, and would just further damage an area already wounded by a clumsy D&C after the miscarriage.

It wasn't only the procedure that appeared brutal to me; the gynecologist had a brutal manner. For one thing, he was a man, which I initially accepted but later realized that my true reaction was intense discomfort. It was incongruous to have a man coldly and clinically discussing the condition of my cervix. I hated the way he winked at me when he told me to "Take your bottom half things off". I hated having an unknown man inserting cold metal instruments inside me and demonstrating the results of his tests to a group of male students. They all stood around, three of them, all male, staring into a microscope that was inserted into my vagina, as I lay with my feet wide apart in stirrups, like some kind of captive animal. I was deeply offended by this. He was treating a very dear and sensitive part of my body as if he temporarily owned it. And I was outraged when he took a biopsy from my cervix without telling me first what he was going to do. The most piercing pain I have ever felt shot through the interior of my body. I screamed, and asked, shocked and terrified, "What have you done to me?" He answered, "Oh be quiet. It doesn't hurt, there aren't enough nerve endings there for it to hurt."

After that I didn't trust him to do anything else to me, and I told him that I felt that there was a psychological reason for my illness, and that I preferred to use gentle methods to heal it. He exploded and told me I was a foolish woman and would undoubtedly die as a result of refusing his surgery. I burst into tears and ran out of his office. How dare he talk to me like that, as if I was nothing, just a body for his skills to work on. I knew that his threat was an attempt to bully me, and one that had no justifiable foundation; the level of dysplasia I had was mild, and had a good chance of getting better without surgical treatment.[1]

Although in Western medicine cervical dysplasia is not considered part of a systemic imbalance, as a doctor of Chinese medicine, I knew that there was another way of looking at the body, one which combined lifestyle and emotional factors with physical dis-ease. I had little faith in the procedures of conventional medicine, because they paid no attention to factors that I was sure were involved in my dis-ease, such as my recent divorce and the way my periods had been recently, and various other factors of which I had only a glimmering awareness. All they looked at was my cervix, and I knew very well that all of me was involved in this aberration from the norm. It seemed poor medicine not to take the other factors into account.

My lack of faith made me very uncomfortable whenever I went for a doctor's visit. It was several years since I had been near a doctor, and in the interim I had been practising acupuncture and living a lifestyle around naturopathic principles. I was shocked when I rediscovered the mind-set that accompanies modern medicine. I would try and talk about my state of mind and how I knew that it was affecting my health and that I was sure that there were less invasive methods of healing that I could use. After all, this was a long way from being a threatening condition. I could afford to take the time I needed to heal more naturally without cutting and cauterizing and traumatizing my body.

No one wanted to listen. They just wanted to do invasive and unpleasant things to me, as fast as possible please, without, it seemed to me, due consideration of the possible outcome. They wanted a quiet compliant patient with no self-awareness. They had stolen my right to my own process of illness and recovery. It seemed obvious to me that if I didn't get the meaning from the message my cervix was giving me, then my body would try again, and I would become sick, perhaps in a different way. It didn't make sense to go ahead and permanently scar my cervix, possibly affecting my ability to carry a child to full term, without trying to understand why my body was behaving in this way.

Each time I had to have a biopsy (I had changed to a different doctor and hospital by this point), the doctor showed no interest in my distaste for the procedure, or for my sense that it might be traumatizing an already upset area.

I knew that the whole thing was tied in with my periods which had been strange for the past few months. My cycle had shortened to 21 days, and I had a very different blood flow. I knew instinctively that something was going on with my womb and that the dysplasia was a symptom of an imbalance that was deeper. I suspected there was an important issue for me to get hold of.

I realized after a while that I really wanted to heal myself. It just didn't feel right to me to go through this surgical business. But I decided I would have to, so I opted for the least invasive remedy: laser treatment. Then a series of interesting synchronicities prevented me from having the treatment. It was delayed and delayed and before the rescheduled date for the treatment, I went to a workshop led by a man who teaches the Native American tradition.

He told me that in the Native American teachings a menstruating woman has the potential to be more psychically and spiritually powerful than anyone, male or female, at any other time. That turned my conditioned pictures of reality upside down. I'd always experienced my period as a time of weakness and difficulty; what on earth was he talking about?

When I asked him specifically about my wounded cervix he asked me a lot of questions and then said that he thought that my problem was rooted in a denial of my femaleness and that he saw that I had negative ideas deep in my unconscious about what it meant to be a woman. He told me to dig a hole in my garden every now and then and speak all the negative thoughts I could think of about the state of being female into the hole, then cover it up so that the earth could transform the energy (just as it transforms waste matter into compost, so it has the capacity to transform our thoughts).

When I went home I tried this technique. I felt pretty silly, and I was glad that no one could see into my tiny garden. I didn't know that I had so many bad feelings about being a woman lurking in my highly-educated feminist mind until I did this exercise. It was painful, and it was very effective.

I started looking at how I behaved when I had my period, and the first thing I saw was that I used tampons. I tuned into my body and in my imagination asked my vagina and cervix what they thought of tampons. "Ugh," they said, unequivocally. "Horrible things." And I thought about it, and realized that maybe there was something important about the blood flowing freely out of the vagina. It occurred to me that the tampons might be irritating my cervix, and I wondered if my initial difficulty with them in my teens hadn't in fact been a wise instinct of my body. I had used tampons without ever thinking about the effect they might be having on me; they were a source of liberation, I thought, one that allowed me to act as if I didn't really have a period.

Aha! I thought. One *that allowed me to pretend I wasn't really having a period.* As I watched that thought, and the thoughts behind it, I began to realize that I had a background belief that my period was something to be ignored and suppressed as much as possible. Suppression was, I knew, one of the main causes of illness and imbalance. Maybe my periods wanted to have a more central place in my life and in my awareness. I began to experiment with that.

If my bleeding started at the weekend, I stopped driving and stayed home, relaxing in my garden. I remember that it was summer and I lay in the sunshine, just experiencing my bleeding. It was interesting to me: I felt so much better if I just lay about and did nothing. If my period started during the working week it was more of a problem, but I would try and rest as much as I could. It was a couple of years before I had the space to really go into what was happening when I was bleeding, but in the beginning it was a major step to allow my period into my life just that much. To sit through the pain instead of reaching automatically for a painkiller, to wear pads instead of tampons and look at my blood and feel the blood coming out of me, to just sit and begin to tune into my bleeding body, to get the first glimmers of a sense of peace that came from just Being, letting go of Doing.

At last I began to feel that I was getting in touch with the root of my problems but the way forward seemed blurry to me. It was clear that in order to heal myself, to become at ease with myself and comfortable in my skin, I had to love my womanliness to a depth that I had not yet plumbed. And in order to do this I had to realize that once again, I had no role models.

I felt very alone. I had a good friend who paid attention to her periods, and her friendship helped me enormously at this time. But I also wanted an older woman as a guide, someone who understood the wholeness of being female in a way that no one around me did. I felt tantalizingly close to this wholeness at times, usually when I was bleeding, but then I would return to my accustomed state of underlying confusion about what it meant to be a woman. In what way was it different from being a man? And how did the menstrual cycle relate to that? I began to wonder about the effect that menstruation had not only on me physically, now that I had realized that it was a time for rest and renewal, but also psychologically and spiritually. What was the meaning of this bleeding time in my overall development, my individuation, and my place in society?

During this time I repeatedly dreamed of a woman who had been bruised and battered. She was very sad, and I would take her in my arms and comfort her. In the dreams I felt shocked at the extent of the cruelty that had been perpetrated on her, and I also saw that she had somehow allowed this damage to take place. I didn't understand why the damage had occurred, but I could hold her in my arms and love her. So I did that, night after night. Sometimes I made love to her. Sometimes I simply held her. Sometimes I just looked at her bruises. I didn't relate to her personally at this time: I had never been beaten like that. Now it is clear that she was a symbol of my wounded woman within, but at the time she was a visitor to my dream-life, and not really a part of "me". Usually she was blonde, which made it harder for me to identify with her personally, because I have dark hair. And maybe she was a visitor, as well as a representation of a part of myself. What was clear was that I loved her and I wanted to heal her.

For me, the wound of being female was a literal wound on the surface of my cervix, and it became clear to me through my dreams and fantasies that my work was to heal the wounded woman within. Doing the exercise of digging the hole in the ground had made me very aware of the largely unconscious negativity that I had towards so much of female reality. I began to look more closely than ever before at what had created that wounding, at what "female reality" actually meant, and at how our society rejected or belittled so much of that. Recovering the beauty and majesty and joy of being female became my task in life.

By allowing my body to be my teacher, by really listening to myself while I was bleeding, I began to understand what the Native Americans were talking about when they stressed the potential power of menstruation.

I began to look at my blood with a tinge of awe rather than fear, disgust, or indifference. By this time I no longer used tampons, so I got to look at my blood properly every month instead of just seeing it on a yucky old tampon. I saw that sometimes it was clear and red, and sometimes darker and clotted. If I really freed up my vision then I could see that it was full of life, full of magic, full of potential. I began to experience a frisson of joy when I thought about bleeding, about being a woman, that there was something, after all, so extraordinarily magical and mysterious about inhabiting a female body. The resentment about being female that I had felt in my teens and early twenties, the feeling that boys had a better deal, faded away and was replaced by a growing sense of wonder at the intricacies and depths and possibilities offered by the monthly cycle.

I began to take time not only to rest but also to meditate and just be with myself when I had my period. I found out that it was a time when I was particularly able to find insight, and that this insight was of a timeless nature. I noticed that my dreams were often very strong, especially towards the end of my period: clear and prophetic. I felt I was tapping into some ancient and vast well-spring of female wisdom, simply by sitting still and listening when I was bleeding. Taking this time out when I was bleeding created a very different relationship with my body. My health improved, my cervix healed, and gradually the bad cramps I had had for most of my menstruating life eased up. My period became a time of pleasure rather than pain.

I was beginning to really love myself. Of course, you can't make yourself do this, just as you can't make yourself love another person. It began to happen, very gradually, and many people came into my life who helped me see more clearly. But the revelation at the beginning was that menstruation is a source of power. This priceless piece of information, coupled with a strong instinct I had about the power of the womb, transformed my deep and largely unconscious lack of self-respect.

This was the information I had needed to give me the confidence to set about healing my own gynecological problems. It inspired me to see if I could feel the power of menstruation if I paid enough attention when I was bleeding. To think of menstruation as a source of power for women completely went against my conditioning, and yet I knew in my heart that it was true. I realized that in the dichotomy between what our culture teaches us, and my gut reaction of "Yes! Of course!" to this ancient wisdom, there was a lot of energy.

When you find the places where a culture splits from a natural truth you have found a key, a way inside the diseases of the culture. I began to understand that the split between the wisdom and power of bleeding that I was perceiving and modern society's attitudes to menstruation lay at the heart of the subjugation and denial of female reality and experience.

CHAPTER FIVE

Menstrual Power and Menstrual Symptoms

Many women suffer from the processes of being female, both physically and psychologically. Our experiences of menarche and menstruation constitute a major part of this experience. Every month, women do something that they are trained to hide and feel ashamed of. Blood stains on clothing are a hideous embarrassment. No one ever says they don't want to come to work or go to the party because they have their period, unless they are feeling really unwell, and then they usually say they have a headache or a stomach ache. And many women experience symptoms every month that they resent and find difficulty in managing or understanding. Our conditioning, our behavior, our attitudes, and our physical and emotional experience, are all interlinked.

When the womb and menstruation are seen merely as uncomfortable biological necessity, women's self-esteem is correspondingly low. We are our bodies, and we can't really love ourselves deep down in the bottom of our hearts if we don't wholeheartedly love our bodies. And you don't love your body if you catch yourself saying, "Oh no, I've got my period."

One of the reasons, of course, that we say such things, is because our lives are planned out in advance. The altered state into which menstruation can take us is not compatible with twenty-first century action-packed life, with running around in the world performing our scheduled and organized tasks. Menstruation is predictably unpredictable. You never know exactly when it is going to come, and sometimes it completely surprises you. Not only is it inconsiderate of timetables and schedules, it is also messy. Hooray! We try to sanitize and order modern life to the degree that we run into danger of there being no life left in us. Periods save us from this doom; they are a wild and basic, raw and instinctual, bloody and eternal aspect of the female, and no amount of "civilization" will change that. Your period is a monthly occurrence in your life that you have in common with all women who have ever lived. Women living in caves twenty thousand years ago, priestesses in pyramids in ancient Egypt, seers in temples in Sumeria, all bled with the moon. The first woman who made fire might well have had her period at the time. Now that's a thought. If menstruation is a highly creative time for women psychically and spiritually, who knows what gifts humankind has been brought by women during their menses. And because menstruation connects us into our wild and instinctual heritage, it has a good deal of raw power contained within it.

The value we place on menstruation has a direct correlation with the value we place on ourselves as women. If we look at the attitudes of matrifocal, earth-centered societies we see a very different relationship with the menstrual cycle. As we saw in Chapter 3, some cultures prize the onset of menstruation and mark it with celebration. In some Native American societies, a menstruating woman's dreams are taken very seriously for their oracular wisdom. In the Tantric tradition, a menstruating woman is considered to be at the height of her power, "a true transmitter of the life force, able to act and respond with true wisdom". [1] It is the loss of contact with this innate wisdom that has led to the distortion of menstrual power into menstrual symptoms.

Both men and women have a collective terror of premenstrual syndrome, evinced by the large number of bad jokes about it. Most women feel victimized by their menstrual symptoms, and powerless to resolve them without using pharmaceutical drugs. And most women have been trained to ignore and suppress information that comes in the form of menstrual symptoms. In order to understand and transform this sorry state of affairs, we need to look at the deep underpinnings of our attitudes, to examine the extent of the fear with which we perceive menstruation.

Anthropological literature abounds with tales of menstrual taboos based on fear of the polluting and dangerous nature of the menstruating woman. When the bodily processes of women and the innate power of menstruation are denied and suppressed, what could be a highly creative energy gets twisted into something "evil". The many taboos about menstruating women show a recognition of power, but usually with a negative interpretation. If a menstruating woman can, as the Talmud warns, cause the death of a man by her mere presence,[2] or, as Pliny tells us, by her touch "blast the fruits of the field, sour wine, cloud mirrors, rust iron, and blunt the edges of knives",[3] then there can be little doubt that something pretty powerful is going on.

Even if we find these beliefs laughable in our rational age, they do show a primitive recognition of the power of menstruation, albeit interpreted from a misogynist perspective. Although these superstitions were part of the weaponry of anti-female propaganda, and were used to restrict and penalize women for their natural bodily functions, at least they did acknowledge that women have power. Nowadays, by ignoring menstruation and suppressing it, we have lost and forgotten this ancient knowledge and have come to believe that our monthly cycle is merely a biological phenomenon.

J. G. Frazer notes in *The Golden Bough* that the same taboos are used for the cloths of menstruating women as for those of holy men and kings.

> The uncleanness, as it is called, of girls at puberty and the sanctity of holy men do not, to the primitive mind, differ materially from each other. They are only different manifestations of the same mysterious energy which, like energy in general, is in itself neither good nor bad, but becomes benificent or maleficent according to its application.[4]

The sacredness and specialness of puberty arises from it being considered a limen, a liminal stage in development where the individual is neither child nor adult, a stage in which the veil between the world thins and the adolescent is vulnerable and porous to the world of the spirit.

In cultures with a benign worldview, this vulnerability is seen as a blessing with the potential for wisdom and transformation. The transition from child to adult is respected and taken seriously. It is considered fundamental to the health of both the individual and the group. The information received by a young Native American during the adolescent vision quest is seen as useful not only for the individual but also for the tribe.

In cultures with a negative worldview, the limen is seen more as a time during which both the tribe and the individual need protection.

Both of these beliefs constitute the root of many of the puberty rituals which take the child away from the rest of the group until he or she is considered to have gone through the limen and emerged as an adult. Usually this emergence is marked by some kind of ceremony. As already noted in Chapter 3, in societies with a benign worldview, the rites of puberty are greeted with joy and celebration, whereas in those with an emphasis on sin and evil and anxiety about bad spirits, the ceremony focuses on casting out demons. In patriarchal societies in particular, a girl's first blood is viewed with fear, suspicion, and even with dread.

Menstruation itself can be viewed as a liminal phase. The woman is in between: she is not pregnant, and neither is she fertile again. She is in a sacred interlude during which she is shedding the past and being renewed before the next opportunity to create human life.

One of the gifts of being female is the access to other worlds that comes during the premenstruum and the time of bleeding. This liminal time opens a woman up to her psychic abilities. Western mechanistic culture prizes the rational and is suspicious of the nonrational: of the intuition, the unseen realms, and the world of the spirit. The Christian church has encouraged us to think of ourselves as separate from God and in need of the intermediary of a priest in order to connect with spiritual realms. This emphasis on rationalism, and the severance from an autonomous relationship with Spirit has served to cut women off from a deep relationship with their menstrual cycle. A great part of women's psychic strength is tied up with the cycles of their bodies, and if we ignore this time and fail to recognize its enormous value then we lose touch with the richness of female experience.

Whether or not this powerful menstrual energy is used in a positive way as with the Nootka and the Yurok, or whether it is uncontrolled and random and is thought to ruin the curing of hams, as with Portuguese villagers,[5] it is nonetheless a form of power. Power is strong energy, and whenever strong energy is not focused and utilized it will act unpredictably. Energy is information; it will always surface somewhere, and if it is not allowed out through the life-force, the creative drive, then it will surface in the body as symptoms or in our emotional lives as relationship problems.[6]

If women access and work with the power of menstruation instead of suppressing it, then this power that so often expresses itself in the form of symptoms becomes free to work in a more harmonious and less disturbing way.

Symptoms wake us up. They draw our attention to the part of the body where they occur. We can't escape our wombs if they are making pain, and we can't ignore the menstrual cycle if it makes us behave differently for a week every month. It is important to remember that symptoms are exactly that: the surface manifestation of a deeper disturbance. They are messages from the body. If you have a healthy lifestyle, a good diet, and enough sleep, and you still have menstrual symptoms, you have to go deeper and ask yourself what your body is trying to tell you. And once a symptom becomes chronic (as in long-term), it is almost always indicative of a deeper issue, because an undisturbed body and psyche will balance itself out, given the right food, water, love, and sleep.

The very aspects of menstruation that we are taught to loathe have within them the seeds of much information. Every time you have a period you are put in touch with the unconscious through your body. So a heavier or lighter flow, more or less pain, and other symptoms, all carry information. Extrapolating the meaning from your period is an individual matter, and involves getting to know yourself and spending time while you are bleeding tuning into whatever is going on.

I found that my menstrual symptoms abated considerably once I started paying attention to my menstrual cycle. I still occasionally get cramps, but nothing like the crippling debilitating pain that I used to get. I never take a painkiller. Lying down with a hot water bottle and entering a relaxed and meditative state of mind eases any discomfort, and it passes quickly. Likewise I still get some mild premenstrual symptoms: a little water retention which I experience as slight breast tenderness, and a tendency to moodiness, depression and elation. This moodiness is actually a sign of the emotional richness of the premenstruum, when we are alive to the full range of our feelings, and this contact with the breadth and depth of our emotions gives the potential for great creativity.

I find that any symptoms that I do experience are a great source of insight into emotional issues to which I need to pay attention. When I have been through a good deal of emotional upheaval, I have found that my periods are a rich opportunity for processing the different feelings that naturally arise during a time of instability and rapid change. I have learnt to trust the process enough to allow these feelings their space when they come up, and during times of change and loss it is not unusual for me to have a spate of weeping at some point during the first day or two of my bleeding. Afterwards I feel lightened, and I know that this emotional release is a part of the moon-time's gift.

Change always brings loss as well as the excitement of the new. It is important to allow grief its place in our lives, and not skate over it. Grief lays the mineral deposits in the psyche that we later mine; our grief is part of the foundation of our wisdom. Most people growing up in the Western world are trained to suppress grief; we have no useful rituals for the dead, no mourning period, no keening. We have tried to erase grief from our emotional repertoire and substituted the expectation of happiness in its place, as if to feel grief were somehow a failing and that to be always happy is the goal of a well-spent life. But that type of happiness is merely bland. It is the so-called happiness of a TV dinner, a beige sofa, muzak piped into supermarkets. True happiness is a joy that wells up from inside the being and is only partly related to external events, and it cannot thrive unless all of its companions – grief and rage and disappointment – are allowed their expression too. Allowing oneself a wide range of emotional expression is the way to be whole.

So women are lucky in this regard, because our periods open us up to our emotional lives and make it harder for us to suppress our feelings. It is the attempt to override this natural mechanism that creates so much disharmony at menstruation, and that lies behind many of the symptoms that women endure.

PREMENSTRUAL SYNDROME

The menstrual educator Tamara Slayton said that PMS should actually stand for PreMenstrual Strength.[7] That is what PMS really is: our female power turned in on itself because patriarchal culture fails to nurture and honor women's reality and women's gifts. When that power is recognized and developed, it becomes clear that what the premenstruum brings is emotional clarity and courage.

During my twenties, I was married for several years. Although we loved each other a lot, it was not a successful marriage; we probably didn't have enough in common to sustain a long-term relationship, or enough maturity to be able to get through the tough times. After a couple of years, I began to suffer from bad PMS and would become really impossible to live with for about a week every month. I found myself hating my husband, finding everything he did irritating. Sometimes I couldn't understand why I was with him, I found him so loathsome. Of course, he wasn't at all, but the suppression of my unhappiness the rest of the month resulted in this outrageous swing into total intolerance during the premenstruum.

He and I colluded in seeing this rage as a biological quirk that had nothing to do with the fact that I was chronically angry with the lack of communication in our marriage. I simply saw it as something that was wrong with me, and I never thought that it might have something useful behind it. After we divorced, and I experienced the relief of being out of a relationship that had been painful for me, I began to see the role my premenstrual anguish had had in destroying the relationship, and a funny little thought crept in: that the PMS was actually a helper, it had helped me to get out. PMS had stopped me from kidding myself. There were always a few days every month when my usual denial was overwhelmed by this deep and uncomfortable knowing that welled up from inside me.

As I began to respect my premenstrual feelings more, my premenstrual anguish eased up and I began to see that it was indeed a friend and ally. If I had a lot of premenstrual symptoms it was a sign to check into my life: what was it I really wanted to be doing, or saying, or experiencing?

Although PMS does involve physical symptoms, for the vast majority of women it is the psychological symptoms which are the most troublesome. Such symptoms include irritability, anxiety, mood swings, depression, hostility, and in severe cases, suicidal or murderous feelings. Eighty percent of women experiencing PMS report that they have increased anxiety and irritability in the days leading up to the onset of bleeding. It is estimated that between one third and one half of all women between the ages of eighteen and thirty-five suffer from PMS, so the incidence of premenstrually-related psychological symptoms affects millions of women.[8]

Let's turn the normal way of looking at these symptoms on its head and instead of seeing them as something unpleasant that should be changed, see them as something potentially useful. What could be useful about being hostile? About being very emotional? About crying and shouting and screaming?

Women are more likely to suffer from PMS if they have children and if they are married.[9] In fact, the harder it is for them to have time alone, the more likely it is that they will experience difficulty with PMS. So it may be that one of the functions of PMS is that through hostility, women repel those around them, and therefore are able to have a little time to themselves. Before I became conscious of my need to spend time alone during the premenstruum, I often experienced a feeling of deep relief when the man in my life took himself out of the house rather than stay around my bad mood. However, it's not quite that simple; some of what comes up during the premenstruum needs to be processed within the context of relationship, not alone.

In order to keep the peace around us, we hold in many of our feelings. And in order to comply with a social norm of unemotional behavior, we even deny those feelings to ourselves. I have no information on the incidence of PMS in cultures that allow and accept emotional expression, but it is interesting to speculate that a woman in Naples who is freer with her feelings during the month might have less need to explode premenstrually than a woman in England where there is a taboo against the outward manifestation of feelings. PMS has the wonderful effect of releasing feelings and opinions that have been locked up for the previous month in the prison of conventional behavior.

I found that when I began to pick up this pattern consciously, I stopped needing to have crazy fights and wild outbursts just before my period; what actually wanted to happen was a clearing up of any relationship difficulties in my life. There were things I needed to say to my partner, to the friend I had that difficult phone call with, to the person I had pretended to be nice to when really I was seething at their thoughtlessness, and so on. Using this time to work on unfinished material, and then to express it, can be very healing for our relationships and can take them into a new realm of connectedness and honesty.

The cleansing aspect of menstruation is important physically, and also psychologically in terms of clarifying and resolving relationships, and not only relationships with other people. It is also a perfect opportunity for clearing up one's relationship with oneself. The tears you didn't cry two weeks ago because you didn't let yourself, come trickling out premenstrually. One of the main causes of illness is unexpressed emotion which has to be expressed somewhere, and so it comes out through the body. Thus PMS is a saving grace for many women in that the lid comes off for a day or two every month, and suppressed emotions are released, lessening the likelihood of them being expressed later through a body symptom.

It also makes sense, given the infinite wisdom and inherent balancing capacity of our bodies, that we would have a time of cleansing and emptying before and as we bleed. The body and the psyche work as one, not separately. As the body releases toxins through the blood, so the psyche releases mental and emotional toxins through the expression of feelings. Often these feelings tend to manifest as anger simply because they have been blocked. Witness the anxious parent whose missing child reappears: her relief soon shifts to anger as the intense feelings she has been holding onto come tumbling out. If feelings are processed as they arise, anger is merely one of a whole range. The issue is whether we allow ourselves the whole range. Most families and most cultures have certain emotions which are less favored and so tend not to be expressed because the individual doesn't identify with them. So we find men who are sure that they are never afraid, women who are convinced that they never feel angry, and many people who think that they are never sad or jealous.

Having a bias against a particular emotion means that emotion is the one that is likely to come out when the defenses are down: during illness, in times of stress, and to varying degrees, in the premenstruum. This is why we don't recognize ourselves and instead say "I turn into a monster just before my period", and seek a physiological reason and a physical remedy. Often there is a physiological reason for which diet and other remedies can be very helpful, but the mind and the body are not separate, and working at a psychological level can do wonders for the health of the whole organism.

Cleansing emotionally always means expression of some type (which does not necessarily involve interaction with others). Many women do this unconsciously because the normal controls fail to operate when they are menstruating. Those who do not may be more likely to break down after childbirth or at the menopause (or at other times of stress), when the lid can no longer be kept on the accumulated tensions of the years.

The connection between the womb and strong outbursts of emotion has long been known. The root of our word *hysteria* is the Greek *hustera*, meaning womb. If we are conscious of the role of menstruation in opening us to emotional expression we can respect the process and work with it; if we deny this process we risk having our feelings erupt violently and painfully in ways which can be damaging to ourselves and to our relationships.

It is interesting that the symptoms of PMS are most severe in women in their thirties and forties.[10] There are many possible explanations for this trend, including the intriguing possibility that PMS is related to individuation. The process of individuation gets going in most people in their thirties and forties, after they have learned to survive in the primary culture. Their psychic energy is then freed up to develop a true individuality. If there is not enough opportunity for this, then the symptoms of midlife crisis may emerge, and one of the ways this manifests is in a desire to get away from the confines of everyday life.

This is similar to the panic, anxiety and overwhelming feelings of PMS. It may be that PMS is a way of allowing a woman to have her individual time for inner work and self-exploration. It is a signal from her body-mind that it requires some attention that it is not getting in the busy round of daily life.

MENSTRUAL PAIN

Menstrual pain has several functions; one of the most obvious is that it shifts our attention to our bodies. It deepens our experience of our bodies and awakens the ability to be aware of the different parts of the body and of bodily sensations. Body consciousness is often an undervalued skill. We are trained in school to think and see and hear, but rarely are we encouraged to feel, with our emotions or our bodies. There is actually a name for this skill of having awareness of inner body sensation: it is called proprioception.

Proprioception is an aspect of inner knowing. Body feelings and intuition are intricately related. We talk of having "gut feelings", of sensing in a very physical way that something was dangerous or wouldn't work out. "It just didn't *feel* right." Being in touch with our bodies enables us to access non-rational information: things we ordinarily couldn't have known. Body feelings are part of our survival instinct and have a warning function.

As a culture we value stoicism and the overriding of the body. We have schedules, appointments, and timetables which are based on industrial efficiency rather than the moment-to-moment needs of the body. We wait until the end of the meeting to empty our bladders, until the end of the day to eat our main meal. We go to work when we have colds, when we have menstrual cramps, when we have a headache. "Not feeling like it" is seen as a pretty lame excuse.

This is very useful training for many situations, but not for everything. And there are certain aspects of being female in which stoicism is exactly the opposite of what is required for successful survival. One of the skills of being a woman lies in being very aware of moment-to-moment bodily needs. Being deeply in touch with her body enables a woman to best nurture her unborn and nursing children. A woman needs to be able to know, and to say, "I need this type of food Now", "I need to rest Now", "I need to drink Now".

The cyclical physiology of women means that their nutritional and rest requirements fluctuate during the month far more than a man's in the equivalent time period. She cannot establish a norm and stick to it come what may. She is a cyclical being, with an ebb and flow of energy.

Getting in touch with that rhythm and finding ways to honor it is a challenge in today's world. Menstrual symptoms pull us back in touch with ourselves. When we have cramps we can't ignore the fact that we are menstruating, and when the pain is really bad it's hard to focus on anything other than the body part that is screaming.

This might sound a bit odd, but this is actually another of the benefits of menstruation. Menstrual symptoms, especially pain, encourage body consciousness by forcing one to experience physical sensations. Women in old age often have an easier time psychologically than men in coping with their bodies, with illness, aging, and pain. One of the reasons may be that they have more of a relationship with their bodies; they are forced into the body by the experience of menstruation and child-bearing. So when their bodies begin to change through the aging process, they are psychologically more accustomed to the fact that bodies change. In many tribes, for example among the Aborigines of Australia, puberty rituals for boys focus on the endurance of pain, whereas this is not considered necessary for girls because nature itself initiates them into their bodies, the experience of physical pain, and the mysteries of life.

Menstrual cramping is often idiopathic; that is, arising from no known organic dysfunction. It is simply a part of menstruation and, in Western medical opinion, doesn't mean that there is anything wrong with the woman. Most women have experienced menstrual pain and many have it every month.

In Chinese medicine menstrual cramps are seen as always being indicative of an imbalance that could be corrected by changes in lifestyle and diet, and/or by taking herbs and having acupuncture. Catching cold is seen as a particular danger for the womb, and that is one of the reasons why heat is often relieving for cramps. The Chinese also recognize that emotional difficulties can give rise to menstrual cramps. Western medicine does not differentiate menstrual pain to this extent and generally prescribes pain-killers only, unless symptoms are severe. Psychologists have begun to develop ways of using psychotherapy to cure body symptoms such as cramps.[11] Bodywork, such as massage, can also be helpful during an attack, and certain yoga poses are also effective. (See Chapter 9 for more information on healing cramps.)

The psychological and emotional causes of menstrual cramps are one of the least understood areas. It is possible sometimes to process your emotional state so that menstrual cramps go away. It all depends on the cause behind the cramping. For example, during one menstrual period I had a lot of pain for several hours in the middle of the first night of bleeding. I knew it wasn't from any physical cause. When I let go of hating it and wishing it would go away, and giving myself a hard time for having it the first place (and feeling guilty because I'm supposed to be so tuned into my periods now that menstruating is all bliss and certainly not painful ... ha!) I realized that I was in pain, that I hurt, and that relief came when I consciously picked up on the feeling of hurt and began to wail and moan. I let all the times when I had felt hurt emotionally in recent weeks come up and I expressed the hurt by yelling and moaning in my bed. I began to feel better and, after acknowledging to myself the source of my hurt, and telling myself that it was okay for me to be sensitive and have feelings, I fell asleep.

My period demands emotional honesty and clarity from me. This includes clearing up the last month's emotional difficulties. We always have relationship issues in our lives, and instances in which we feel hurt or slighted in some way. Sometimes these are well within the bounds that we can handle, and our resilience prevents wounds from going deep. But there are times when we do feel vulnerable. Usually we protect ourselves from this by deciding that it doesn't really matter, we don't care anyway, and it's no good going through life being so sensitive.

But there is a part of us that does care, that cares very deeply about our own pain, and the pain of others. And if we block off from our own pain then ultimately we block off from the pain of others.

Menstrual pain puts us in touch with our feelings of being hurt, and by really expressing this hurt we can process the pain. By this I mean we can release it by acknowledging it. Life is a process of gaining self-knowledge. Symptoms give us information. If you don't express your pain verbally or in some other conscious and creative way then it may be expressed unconsciously through the body as pain. Menstruation is a wonderful opportunity for women to process hurt feelings, rage, and frustration.

Menstrual pain can be really awful. As with labor pains, we obscure reality if we try to imagine that it doesn't really hurt, and for some women, the pain that comes with menstruation has an excruciating and seemingly unbearable intensity. But ut can still be processed and worked through.[12]

There is a similarity between the pain of labor and the pain of menstruation – both are caused by uterine contractions (unless there is a physical problem causing the menstrual pain, such as endometriosis). When a woman menstruates, she is laboring to give birth to herself. Menstruation is the rebirth of the woman; it occurs instead of the onset of pregnancy, and means that she is free, for the next month at least, of sharing her body with another; free of the responsibility of motherhood and the weight (literally) of the unborn child.

MENSTRUATION AND PHYSICAL RENEWAL

Most women, when left to their own devices, report that they like to take it easy on the first day or two of their periods.[13] The natural inclination to rest and be still during menstruation is an opportunity for physical renewal. Physically, bleeding is a form of elimination and is therefore a cleansing for the body. Through cleansing and retreat the woman becomes revitalized. The debilitating symptoms that arise at the time of menstruation are often a message from the body to *stop!* Often, simply lying down and having a rest will ease cramps. Lie down and rest and listen to the body wisdom that is trying to come through you. Let your body take this natural break in the month to rest and rebuild. We need to relearn the ancient knowledge that menstruation is an important juncture in the month. It is a built-in time for rest, retreat and renewal.

Often our long-term, deep healing comes through the very simple: more rest, more love, doing the work we love; going back to basics. It is this level of healing that I address in this book. Imagine how healing it is to be alone, quiet and undisturbed, able to rest and retreat for at least a few hours while you are bleeding and perhaps also for a day or two before the bleeding starts. That's all; it is really very simple. We need to be supported in following the wisdom of the body which slows down and beckons us to focus internally during the bleeding time. We need not to work, not to relate, not to be under any pressure to be anything other than ourselves. We need to allow our natural wisdom and creativity to emerge in this quiet space in the month, to emerge in its own time, in its own way. The wisdom of women is linked to the womb and the power of the womb is the power of cycles and of gestation. Allowing time, allowing emptiness, allowing not-doing – these are all keys to health for women.

It's very healthy to shed a skin; it allows the detritus of the past to be sloughed off, and then the new, clean, smooth skin shows up on the surface and we are renewed. The blood that was a part of us is now gone, leaving the womb cleaned out and ready for the next month. This cycle is beneficial to our overall health. A friend of mine once said that he always thought that women lived longer than men because they menstruate, and some tribes share this belief.

Developing a love for and a connection with the power of menstruation also means developing a love for and a connection with the process. It won't work if the relationship you have with your bleeding is a theoretical one. You have to change your behavior in order for the power to begin manifesting in a positive way. The power backfires on us if we don't honor our bleeding and develop a conscious relationship with it, if we don't pick up the messages our bodies send us. Cultivating a loving attitude towards one's whole cycle is crucial; this attitude is the metaskill behind menstruating with awareness.

At times, and especially at the beginning, negative feelings will surface and want to be expressed. Don't hold them back. You may need to scream with rage at the inconvenience of it, at the messiness, at the pain. But keep behind that an attitude of loving yourself, loving your body, loving the reality of being female, and gradually the balance will begin to shift. It is fundamental to developing the skills of being a woman to trust the process that is inherent within us and that has been denied us because we have been indoctrinated into a male reality.

THE FOUR PHASES OF MENSTRUATION:
THE CYCLE WITHIN THE CYCLE

From my meditations during my periods, and from discussions with other women, I have discovered that there is a cycle within the monthly cycle: a cycle of energy and awareness that exists within the period itself. This is the pattern I have uncovered:

Phase One : The Preparatory Phase

Phase One is often called PMS, but really something much deeper that being a bitch is going on here. This is the time to clear up any relationship issues (given that you feel able to do this) and to complete any unfinished tasks from the previous month. Then you use the energy of the premenstrual time to prepare logistically for your retreat, and that organizational urge signals that menstruation is imminent.

Phase Two : The Major Bleeding and Release Phase

Phase Two begins at an emotional level shortly before the first blood flow, and continues as we experience and release feelings and information from the near or distant past, up to and including the first day or so of bleeding. The intensity of this phase depends on many factors: current state of well-being, amount of time and space available for processing the emotional material, and many other individual and time-specific factors such as age, predisposition, diet, location, and work-load.

Phase Three : The Emptiness Phase

Phase Three segues on from Phase Two after the emotional catharsis completes, and is characterized by an experience of emptiness. This can last for several days, or for only hours, depending on, yet again, a myriad of factors.

Phase Four : The Wisdom Phase

Phase Four arises toward the end of bleeding, and is usually only felt if you have allowed Phases Two and Three to occur fully. Phase Four is a remarkable gift: a period of clarity and receptiveness, in which new information comes in, both personal and collective, which helps you plan for the future.

(These four phases are discussed in more detail in Chapter 7.)

THE MENSTRUAL JOURNEY

The journey of each period begins with a sense of uncomfortable fullness before the period starts. This fullness is familiar to almost all women, and is as much a psychic condition as it is physical. It is irritating and one becomes irritable. Then there is the stage of release, followed by a time of nothingness, after which the psychic and physical arc of the period completes itself with a sense of deep renewal. At this point we reach the other side of that initial irritation, and experience a sense of effortless peace and well-being. This arc is very similar to all creative processes, including giving birth.

This journey is also a spiritual journey, and follows the same pattern as the classical path to spiritual awakening: depression and a sense of meaninglessness leads to a search for inner truth which results in growing authenticity and the expression of pent-up feelings. This release into truth is followed by an experience of emptiness leading to a sense of oneness-with-everything and a deep understanding of the meaning of life.

Every time you menstruate you have the opportunity to deepen psychologically and spiritually. In the next chapter we will look more closely at the relationship between menstruation and the spiritual lives of women.

CHAPTER SIX

The Sabbath of Women: Spirituality and Menstruation

Women give, and in order to give they have to take in. They do this by first emptying and cleansing, and then by renewing their connection to the source. This is the function of menstruation.

About three years after I began taking menstruation seriously and changing my behavior during my periods (which coincided with a time of emotional upheaval, spiritual searching, psychological work and shamanic practice), I had an experience which gave me some crucial information about the nature of menstrual traditions in ancient matrifocal societies.

It was part of a transformation of my life that had begun a year earlier when I let go of virtually everything I owned and connected with, including my medical practice, my home, and my country of origin. I felt driven by some huge force to clear myself of everything that contributed to my conditioned view of life and of myself.

I then entered a period of bliss. I was in love with everyone and everything and experienced life as an ever-opening kaleidoscope of magic and beauty. I had many wonderful experiences of being at-one with everything, of merging with my lover totally, of experiencing the universe as pure love.

After six months of this I entered the territory of the shadow: I became very sick while traveling in Nepal, and along with the illness came a descent into a deep depression. I was physically blasted by the illness and stayed in bed at first, and then chiefly indoors and in a safe place for several months. I was beset by intense and uncontrollable fear and shaken to the core by the whole experience. Several times I completely lost faith in the flow

. my life and in my spiritual connection. I felt abandoned and close to destroyed, and by what? I hadn't a clue. The ideas that I was holding onto about who I was and was not were preventing me from really being myself. I knew that I wanted to write, that it was vitally important for me to allow my creativity to have expression, but I lacked confidence, and was fighting demons of self-criticism and distrust.

The recovery period was slow. When feeling optimistic I perceived the illness as a major purification, and it felt as if my body had been rewired in order to handle a new frequency of energy. When feeling that I would never fully recover (my energy level was unpredictable for a year after the initial onslaught), I worried that my nervous system had been permanently damaged and feared for the health of my heart, which raced at the slightest opportunity.

While I was putting myself back together, feeling like a newborn foal on wobbly legs, and gradually finding that I could cope with the world again, I had, out of the blue, the strongest experience of the whole transformation period.

I awoke at about 4 a.m. from a dream which propelled me into a series of experiences of a woman named Hathor living in ancient Egypt. I was used to having past-life experiences, but this had a different quality. It was as if I was allowed to enter Hathor's reality, and that she and I were (and are) intimately and intricately and eternally connected, but that we are also clearly different people. She is startlingly alive to me, and as a result of "feeling" her, I no longer experience time in only a linear framework.

Hathor lived (or lives) at a time when patriarchal ideas were just beginning; a time when the Goddess was still revered, a time when women had their own temples and their own rituals, a time when women's wisdom was respected and encouraged.

I was astonished by the experience of making this connection with her, but also settled by it. I began to calm down, to have a sense of my direction, and, at last, to take my writing seriously. I began a dialogue with her which I usually wrote down as it came through and one day, several months later, I asked her what the women of her time did when they menstruated.

"When a woman felt her time coming, she would bake food for the family, put some in a bag for herself, and then walk up to the moon house. This house was outside the town on the top of a hillside which had on one side been eroded into a cliff by the river. The house overlooked the town to the north, the river to the east, and the gentle slope of the hills to the west, and then the desert beyond and behind, on the far side of the fertile plain.

During the walk up the hillside the woman would begin to let go her attachment to her family and her life and its obligations down in the town. She would already be entering the dreaminess of her moon-time when she arrived at the top of the hill and walked down the path through the simple garden. She was greeted by the housekeeper, an older woman past menstruating age who kept the hearth of the house. She would give the housekeeper a small amount of money and go inside and take a bed in the dormitory.

She would speak quiet words of greeting to the other women, but this was not a time for gossip or chat, or even serious talk. This was a time to go inside, to be alone, even when amidst others. Occasionally, when a woman felt particularly moved to seek the wisdom within, or in need of great cleansing, she would go off alone into the desert for her moon.

The moon house was very simple. One large room full of beds, a shrine room for contemplation, and a platform overlooking the river on which they ate the simple meals they had brought with them. From the bedroom the windows faced east and had beautiful views of the river and of the mountains beyond. There were no windows to the north and west and therefore no view of the town or the fields. The walls were built of a light-colored stone, and the beds were spaced well apart from each other. The shrine room was dark, in the center of the house, and in it was a statue of Isis and black cushions on which to comfortably sit.

The atmosphere in the house was restful, peaceful, uncluttered. A place to let go. Often women would be heard weeping to themselves, or some other release. This was accepted as part of the moon and was not interfered with in any way by the other women. If a woman became particularly distressed she could go to the housekeeper, but it was taboo to disturb others. Each respected the others' going inside. A time when women had no responsibility to care for others – the necessary balance to the role of caregiver."

Six months later, while meditating on the first day of my period, I found myself in a deep trance in which I received the following advice:

Guidelines for Menstruating Women

Stay still inside and let the blood flow out.

See your womb as an opening flower, full of fierce pink light, sending out a special sweet rosy energy into the world, which cleans and nourishes.

Let the beauty blood spill onto the earth.

Trust the wisdom of the body's cycle. Honor it. Go with what your body wants to do.

Take gentle peaceful exercise, in quiet places. Listen to slow flowing water, the tinkle of a fountain in a stone-flagged square.

Take a slow look, and a slow movement. Turn your head gently.

Stroke yourself. Let all your movements be soft and serene.

Speak with gentleness. No fights.

Eat simple food: grains and vegetables and broth.

Nothing too rich or sweet or milky.

Drink pure water, savoring the taste and clearness.

Go inside, deep inside, and allow any murkiness to be
seen, and to flow out. A time of clearing out and of
taking in.

Be alert to information for the coming month.

Relax. Be soft. Slow down.

Open your womb, your thighs, your knees, your
ankles, your toes. Open your heart. By opening, let go,
let the blood flow.

This advice profoundly affected me and sent me deeper into
my experience of the menstrual mysteries. I found that following
these guidelines took me into my center and put me in touch with
a wellspring of wisdom and knowledge. This affirmation of the
concept that menstruation is a time of power gave me the
confidence to question more intently our contemporary attitudes,
not only to menstruation, but to cycles in general.

Feeling this new sense of personal power and wholeness set
me thinking about the nature of modern life and how difficult it
is for us to live in such a centered and healing way, how hard it
is for us to honor the natural cycles of our bodies, and just how
far we have gone from the wisdom of these ancient voices.

MENSTRUATION AS SABBATH

The ancient Babylonian word for Sabbath, *sabbatu*, comes
from *Sabat*, and means heart-rest. In Babylon it was a day of rest,
when the goddess Ishtar was said to be menstruating. Travel,
work, and eating cooked food were prohibited for everyone on
this day, as they were for menstruating women in many cultures.[1]
Cuneiform tablets from the fourth dynasty of Ur, dating from the
third millennium B.C.E., tell us that in Sumer the times of the new

moon and full moon were devoted to ritual observance. Likewise, the Jewish Sabbath originally occurred at the new moon and full moon; it was later extended to each quarter of the moon.[2] These distant days of rest, linked to the moon and to menstruation, were the origin of the modern Jewish Sabbath and Christian Sunday.

These days, few people take even one day a month to really rest. In general, Western culture is obsessed with the Doing mode of living. We only value ourselves if we are doing something. and we think that people who don't do very much are less valid members of society. We are oriented toward productivity and the accumulation of wealth and possessions rather than toward the accumulation of wisdom, spiritual strength, and self-knowledge.

This continual Doing does not lead to happiness or well-being, and we all know the relief of being on holiday and not having to Do anything. Now, obviously, it would unbalance us in the other direction if we all laid down our tools and decided to just Be, but maybe we could use a little more stillness and unpressured hanging-out times in our lives, and I don't mean sitting in front of the television watching people kill each other and cheat on their spouses. I'm thinking more of sitting in front of a tree, or a lake, or the sea, and just Being.

There was a good deal of value in the old idea of the Sabbath: empty time with no labor, devoted to prayer and contemplation. As the industrial age built up steam, powered by the Protestant work ethic, the Sabbath fell out of favor and the old taboos against working on one day of the week disappeared. This can only be adding to the stress and pressure of modern life. Our bodies and our minds need to take time out, they need a periodic rest, and our spirits need to be nurtured, they need some time devoted purely to the spiritual life. The lack of Sabbath may be why so many people get colds and flu: that is the only way they can have a Sabbath, a rest from continual Doing.

In many parts of America, the only way you can tell it's Sunday is that the beaches and parks are more crowded, the Sunday paper is on sale, and there is less traffic in the downtown areas. Other than that, everything is the same. All the shops are open, and most services are available. And the television never sleeps.

If you are always racing about, doing this and that, always running behind yourself, when do you have time to really feel your feelings? When do you have time to reflect upon why you reacted so strongly when a colleague said they hated animals in the house, why your husband is annoying you so much at the moment, why you hate wearing red, why the thought of your mother coming over for lunch fills you with dread. You might have quick ideas about what these things mean, you may just push them aside and keep running, but you won't understand them and heal the difficulties in your life if you don't have some quiet time.

A woman's moon-time is the obvious time in her cycle to take a break from Doing, and to just sit and be, to sit and bleed. It is a natural time for opening to the spiritual realms, and for doing the work of knowing and understanding the self that can only happen in empty, still, quiet time.

In the Jewish tradition, the first day of each month (which would have been the day of the New Moon before we went solar, traditionally the time of menstruation) is a women's holiday, called Rosh Chodesh (head of the month). This holiday is being reclaimed by some Jewish women. This was a ritualized acceptance of the desire for women to have a break when they are bleeding.

Peaceful time is very useful for relationship problems, and sitting quietly for a few hours can do wonders for restoring perspective. Many squabbles and fights arise from our over-stimulated adrenal glands, which are for many people continually fired up on all cylinders, fighting through the traffic to get to work, dealing with work pressures and deadlines, coping with a family as well as a job, and then the television is on all night screaming away at you, and there is no peace.

We have become so used to this pressurized existence in the Western world that many people have forgotten how to sit still. It seems boring because we have grown accustomed to continual external stimulus. But there is an inner life as well as an outer life, and that inner life, the life of the psyche, is very precious and is the wellspring of our creativity, of our gift to the world. Ultimately we may not give anything of great value without nurturing this inner life. And it needs quiet time to grow and develop.

We can relearn how to be in the rhythm of stillness again; we knew how to once, when we were babies and small children and went from bursts of rapid activity to moments of stillness and sleep and then back into activity again. We need to give ourselves time: time to absorb change, time to let ourselves take in everything around us; not taking life as a whistle-stop tour in which we have to grab as much as we can before we are thrown off the train. We have to give ourselves time to get in touch with stillness again, by practicing sitting still. Many people have the experience of going on holiday and not knowing what to do with themselves for the first few days with all that open and unstructured time. And then after three or four days they remember how to just be, and by the time they are really loving it, it's time to come home again. If we had more time like this in the regular routine, perhaps life would become less of a pressure and more of a pleasure.

By taking menstruation as the natural time for stillness and quiet in a woman's life, we can begin to relearn the rhythm of sitting in peace with ourselves, and then we can begin to reap the benefits of a closer relationship with our inner beings.

Menstruation can be a deeply grounding and centering time, in which a woman is naturally put directly in touch with her center of gravity: her womb. Thus there is actually a greater capacity for stillness at this time; for listening, for receiving from the cosmos. The awareness that is available to us during menstruation cannot come into our consciousness if we are rushing about fulfilling the exterior demands of our everyday lives.

Sitting still and being centered are prerequisites in all spiritual traditions for the development of wisdom. Menstruation is a natural time for women to meditate and make contact with the divine, within and without. When the body is still, the mind also becomes still and then the spiritual wisdom that exists at a deeper level of consciousness is free to come to the surface of our awareness.

Discovering Who you Really Are & What you Really Want

Menstruation is a door into oneself. Traditionally, girls entering puberty knew to watch for a vision of their future when they had their first period. It was recognized that menarche is a door into adulthood, where visions of one's life are available so that correct choices can be made in order to follow one's heart's desire and fulfill one's destiny and deepest dream. Likewise, the monthly bleeding is a doorway into the forthcoming month, and sometimes, when the energy is very strong, into a longer period of one's life.

By tuning into yourself during bleeding and opening up to this gateway, you allow information in the psyche to emerge into consciousness: information about what you truly want and need. This is so valuable, and yet it is an ability of ours that we tend to dismiss. We go to career counselors and psychotherapists for the very information that we alone possess. A skilled helper will work to enable you to unravel the knotted skein of desire within you, but it is also possible to do this alone by connecting with your body rhythms in a deep way.

When you have your period, if you allow yourself some quiet time, you will find that ideas and knowledge and information will begin to come to you. It will usually come in the form of a knowing, that can slip away if not caught and held onto. Watch out for the early morning when you first wake up. There is often juicy information around then. Keep paper and a pen next to your bed to jot ideas down.

You may also find that you begin to receive information about other people. My experience has been that in opening up to the menstrual mysteries, I have also opened up to an ability to be intuitive in a way that allows access to the collective mind, where information about anyone and anything is available if you have the psychic awareness to pick it up.

From what I have read about cultures in which the time of menstruation was regarded as a time of power for women, I suspect that women have a particularly strong capacity to enter this level of universal information. Either this capacity is strongest during menstruation, or menstruation is the best time to develop this awareness, perhaps because then the body and mind are relatively still. It may be that anyone who enters contemplative mode for long enough would begin to manifest this ability to channel information, and that it is simply because menstruation offers such a perfect opportunity to be still and inner that it produces this effect. However, there is such a dominant archetype of the female medium in today's culture, that for now, at any rate, it appears that mediumistic abilities are more the domain of women than of men.

THE DEVELOPMENT OF WISDOM IN WOMEN

A woman who uses her time of bleeding to develop her inner life, and therefore her self-knowledge, begins, over time, to become wise. Life is the teacher of wisdom, and it is life experienced with awareness that creates wisdom in the elderly. But children can also be wise. There is a level of awareness available to humans that is simply wise, and we can foster the ability to enter that level. One of the keys to this simple wisdom seems to be to really know ourselves in the moment, and to act without unnecessary inhibition. This is why children are sometimes more open to wisdom than most adults.

Living is, in part, a quest to understand how to be oneself, a truly differentiated individual, within a society that demands certain inhibitions in order to maintain harmony in the whole. Navigating one's way through this terrain of personal desire versus collective demand is the task of the adult, and the ideal is for the mature years to be an expression of all that is best about both: to be a developed individual – to "know thyself" – and at the same time to be a worthy citizen of the world who is able to give wisdom and knowledge back into the soup of the collective.

MENOPAUSE AND THE ARCHETYPE OF THE CRONE

In later life, the urgency of fulfilling personal desire decreases. For men and women, changes in hormones and the completion of certain life tasks, such as raising a family and becoming established in the world, allow the desire nature to subside. Without the monthly surge and wane in hormones, a woman's sexual longing and desire to reproduce calm down, and the desire mechanism in general becomes less strident. As a society, we need post-menopausal women whose main attention is no longer focused on getting what they want but has moved on toward giving the accumulated wisdom of their years back to the world.

The Celts said that a post-menopausal woman was wise because she now kept the precious blood within her. I speculate that a post-menopausal woman is wise because she has menstruated for thirty or forty years and during that time she was a gatherer of wisdom. Now, having gathered it in, she sits on it and lets it build, fortified by the experience of her lifetime. A lifetime of garnering wisdom every month leads to a wise old age. The perpetual round of the menstrual cycle tunes a woman into the pulse of the earth and the rays of the moon. It gives her the knowing, in her body, of the cyclical nature of all life. Now that women can realistically expect to live for at least twenty to thirty years past menopause, as a culture we have a potentially vast resource of wise women, if we would only use it.

The current obsession with staving off menopause through the use of hormone replacement therapy misses the point that there is an inherent value in ceasing to menstruate. Perhaps women feel the need to prolong their menstrual experience because they never really had it; because they spent their periods pretending that nothing was happening. Maybe the desire to continue to bleed is actually an unconscious attempt to complete that part of life.

Menopausal women speak of their sense of loss of a cycle never properly lived. Their periods end and then they realize, too late, what a gift was held in their monthly bleeding. As with any grief, it is the unacknowledged and unlived aspect that is often the most painful. When someone dies with whom you have a lot of unresolved or unexpressed feelings, things you wanted to say but didn't, love or anger never clearly expressed, there is often a very deep pain. Likewise with menstruation: it is the unacknowledged part of it that causes the most painful aspect of the grief of menopause. If you have given yourself time to enjoy bleeding and to reap the benefits of conscious menstruation, then the menopause becomes more a welcomed passage than the loss of a womanhood you never really had. This is, in part, why women crave their youthfulness in contemporary Western culture and why they spend billions of dollars to avoid looking like who they really are: post-menopausal women.

And of course, the archetype of the old, wise woman, the crone, is not valued in Western society. The development of the patriarchy involved a systematic destruction of the power of old women. The witch-hunts of the Inquisition and subsequent suppressive movements were frequently aimed at old women who knew how to heal and how to assist at births and deaths. (The crone – in Greek myth characterized as Hecate – stands at the crossroads of life and death and can help souls on their way in and out of corporeal existence.)

In other cultures and in other times, wise women have been venerated and integrated into society. A look at the marriage ceremony is a stark example of how the crone has been sidelined, ejected from our conscious lives. In traditional Breton weddings the three phases of the bride's life were celebrated: impersonating her first by a little girl (the maiden), then by the mistress of the home (the mother), and then by an old grandmother (the crone). These three phases are an expression of female wholeness, mirroring the waxing, full, and waning phases of that emblem of the feminine, the moon.[3]

In modern weddings we still have the maiden represented as the flower girl or bridesmaid, and the mother represented as the matron-of-honor, but the crone figure is no longer present. She has been relegated to an unconscious position, no longer given a ceremonial place in our most crucial social and personal ritual.

In contemporary society, we see the maiden everywhere; she

is the archetype of female splendor paraded across magazines and movie screens. The mother has some value, and is even, in a limited aspect, revered as Mother Mary in contemporary religion. But the crone appears nowhere. She is the hidden archetype of this culture, all her power hidden in the underbelly of our lives.

We have become collectively terrified of aging. As a direct corollary, we seem to pay less and less attention to what it takes to gain true wisdom, as opposed to the glib form of information overload that too often passes for knowledge today. A culture that reveres youth over the wisdom of age is an immature culture, and it is therefore no wonder that our supposedly civilized society is not in the least bit mature, but is in fact riddled with addictions, the widespread misuse of resources, and endemic violence.

As the baby boomer generation ages, we may well see the elderly given the same amount of attention that teenagers had in the sixties, young parents in the eighties, and middle age in the nineties. Perhaps we will see old age become the most hip and lively place to be. We may eventually see a shift in favor of old age, because that generation will still be the wealthiest and the most influential by sheer force of numbers. But this is a strong tide to try and turn, and it could be frittered away in an obsession with using pharmaceutical drugs and cosmetic surgery to keep us all looking strangely youthful.

Women themselves have to take back the power of their cronedom and own the reality, the pain, and the glory of the aging process. The world needs centered, grounded, bullshit-free old women, who are liberated from personal insecurities and petty anxieties.

ALTERED STATES OF CONSCIOUSNESS

For women involved in spiritual practice and creative work, menstruation gives an opportunity for increased access to non-ordinary states of awareness. Many women experience difficulty in thinking in a focused way during or just before the period (as they also do after giving birth, often for several months). The energy that is usually available for focused thought is diverted into other areas, and the woman experiences a more diffuse state of awareness.

This is the state in which creative insights can sneak in, when lateral thinking is easiest, when we can let go of our accustomed perceptions and attitudes. Input from other dimensions is more readily available. Activities of a visionary and intuitive nature have added energy and possibility at this time: dreaming, receiving information about the coming month, gaining awareness of psychological patterns, receiving teachings from spiritual guides, experiencing psychic connections with others. I have had many experiences of prophetic dreams during menstruation. I have found that the last couple of days of my period tend to be the strongest for precognition. It seems that the premenstruum and the first couple of days are mainly occupied with cleansing and processing, and then the way is open to receive wisdom and insight. Just as at menarche girls seek visions for their adult lives, so one can look for information about the coming month during one's period.

Monica Sjoo says that "shamanism – an ecstatic lunar cult – relies on the natural descent into body-consciousness that menstruation brings each month".[4] The descent of the shaman is so similar to the monthly descent of the woman into herself, that it seems likely that the moon-time is a natural opportunity to do shamanic practices and seek altered states of consciousness. "At menstruation, when the body passes its blood-food, a woman often feels an ingathering of her energy and feelings to a deeper center below the threshold of consciousness." [5] The shamanic journey may have its origins in the psychic journeys of menstruating women. Similarly, Alaskan and Siberian shamans talk of going to the moon.

The death and rebirth motif of menstruation parallels shamanic experience. The feeling of death at the onset of menstruation; the sense, particularly during the premenstruum, of going down into the mire and the darkness of ourselves: this descent is an essential part of shamanic transformation. The shaman descends, faces death, and through courage and determination, returns to his or her people with special gifts of healing and wisdom.

The fear of death in our non-spiritual culture is linked to the denial of menstruation. In pre-industrial society, women menstruated together around the time of the new moon. Moon-dark is a two-day period of time before the new moon when there is no moonlight at all. Before we see the light of the new moon we experience a temporary death, a darkness. Menstruation coincides with this; it marks the death of a potential life. It is a release of the layers built up during the month, the layers of physical blood, and also the psychic debris and emotional clutter of the previous four weeks.

Like the shaman, the menstruating woman has been seen as somehow mysteriously closer to the sacred aspect of nature than other human beings. In the Indian cult of Shakti-worshippers, the yoni and its red flow are prized and adored. "In Shaktism the menstrual taboo is broken down and the menstrual fluid is regarded as sacred and becomes the object of veneration. A menstruating woman is placed in a special category during ritual practice. Her energy at this time is said to be different in quality, and the rhythm that occurs in her body appears to be related in a mysterious way to the processes of nature…. The monthly efflorescence of woman in her cycle in rhythm with the lunar cycle creates a body consciousness which is related to the processes of the universe." [6]

Imagine how it would be if we were raised to think of our blood as divine, as magical, as precious. Experiencing the beauty and intense spirituality of bleeding can dramatically change a woman's relationship with herself. While meditating during my period I have seen my womb as a golden chalice spilling forth a constant stream of white light, intermingled with the red blood of life. Visions such as this can have the effect of permanently altering and healing the negative images of the female that we have been fed. This heals us, body and the soul, from the wounds of ignorance and misogyny.

PART THREE

RITUALS AND RECOMMENDATIONS

Chapter Seven

Conscious Menstruation: First Steps

If you decide you want to find out more about yourself and about being a woman, if you decide to really enter into your power as a female being, if you decide you want to menstruate in a self-loving, self-accepting way, there is one very simple step to take that will get you started. When you have your period, take some time to yourself. This is the starting place that allows all the benefits of menstruation to come to the surface, instead of being buried, as they have been for so long, under a heavy blanket of denial, suppression, and ignorance.

We live in such an extroverted society that it is often hard for us to imagine how we would actually manage to find some time to be in silence. Then we wonder if, having found the time, we could stand the aloneness and quiet, so acculturated are we to noise and stimulus.

The best recommendation I can make is that you try it, and to tell you the story of what happened to me when I followed the energy of my periods and began to let retreats happen to me in a very natural way. Bear in mind that my journey was an extreme one, and I am not suggesting, by telling my story, that you need to go and live out in the wilds and be by yourself for days at a time. You may choose to do that at some point, and I do think that such experiences are wonderfully enlivening and strengthening, but what may work better for you is to take my story and use the spirit of it as a starting point to stimulate your own way of finding a retreat and balance space.

As I mentioned earlier in the book, when I learned about the powerful and sacred nature of menstruation from the Native American teachings, I began to spend time being simply quiet, especially on the first day of bleeding. As time went on I felt an increasing need for solitude at that time, and I came to realize that for me, at least fifty percent of my PMS was a plea to be alone to process the previous month. (The other fifty percent needed to be processed in relationship to others, not alone). I was beginning to see that when I gave myself sufficient peaceful time, something very interesting began to happen toward the end of the bleeding, and I was looking for a chance to explore this further.

Then I fell in love with a man who had a house in a quiet and beautiful spot on the shore of a lake in the mountains, and as this house was empty most of the time I was free to use it whenever I wanted. It felt particularly fitting to my task that the house was situated on a wild and peaceful part of the shore of Lake Tahoe, a huge lake sacred to the Native Americans.

I was in my early thirties at this time, and like many young women I still had a lot to discover about myself. I also had various aspects of my emotional past that needed to heal. And because of the time in which I was living, I had a lot to discover about being truly comfortable with being a woman. I wanted to find out more about the mysterious power that I knew was associated with menstruation and from which women had clearly become distanced in modern society.

I began to fully retreat when I had my period, being quiet and alone, sitting on the earth in the sunshine with lizards and blue jays for company, with the wind and the moon and the sun, the ripples and the colors on the lake my guides and entertainers. I wandered in the vast forest behind the house, and spent days without seeing a soul. I journeyed inside my psyche and would find myself suddenly in tears at something long forgotten, an event from my childhood or adolescence. My period became a time when I found I was particularly able to open up to my inner life and release emotions.

I noticed that after the first few days of bleeding I would go very still and quiet for a day or so and seemingly nothing would be happening: an empty space after the weeping and remembering. Then as my period ended there would be several hours of clarity in which I would be particularly creative and also open to information about the future; usually the coming month, but sometimes reaching beyond that.

This pattern continues for me, some ten years after I first

discovered it, although usually it is less intense these days. Much of the deeply held psychological clutter has been released. I feel more up-to-date with myself so there is less to let go of, usually just anything I have held onto from the preceding month.

I don't have a daily meditation practice. I prefer to adjust my inner and contemplative time to my own impulses. Often when I have my period I go into a quiet, solitary, and meditative space for three or four days, and then much less the rest of the month. This feels like a very natural rhythm to me, and that's why I think of the bleeding time as the Sabbath of women.

PLANNING YOUR RETREAT

But how can we create sacred time and space for ourselves in modern life? For most of us this is a problem for which we continually seek to create a variety of solutions. Countless women have told me that they wish they had access to a moon-lodge or equivalent, some house that was just for menstruating women to go and be left alone. There are places where women are creating such havens, but in the absence of these being a regular part of most people's lives, here are some suggestions for how you can go into retreat for yourself.

Plan ahead for when you think your period is due. Perhaps, like me, your periods are not precisely regular: I have a twenty-six to twenty-eight day cycle. If this is the case, make a note of when it is most likely to come, and plan to be flexible around these dates. Plan to do as little as possible during that time and for at least three days after, meaning that about five or six days will be planned for, although only three or four of these will actually be a time when you will be menstruating, depending on the length of your bleeding time.

You will have a month's warning of when your bleeding time is likely to come, so you can plan your social life, meetings, appointments and so on around it. I have found that a good deal of the perceived difficulty around taking time out comes out of our cultural indoctrination to make light of our periods. Once that shifts, so does one's ability to claim and create time to oneself.

In Chapter 5 I outlined the Four Phases of Menstruation. Here is a more detailed description of these phases that occur within the period itself. Understanding and feeling these shifts in energy and emotion will help you to manage your time to maximize the potential of your moontime.

A MAP OF THE MENSTRUAL TERRAIN

Phase One : The Preparatory Phase

You may find yourself entering a different state of awareness a few days before the bleeding starts. I often notice a dreaminess beginning about two days before my period but I don't usually feel the strong need to withdraw until I begin to bleed. Women really differ in this and for some women it is during the week before their period that they want to withdraw, and then when they begin to bleed they feel like being out in the world again. You have to tune into what is right for you.

In the day or two before I begin to bleed, I usually stop wanting to drive. As much as I can, I follow that feeling and organize my life so that driving is at a minimum. If I have to go somewhere I minimize the amount of driving, by not doing any unnecessary errands or social calls. If I'm with someone else I ask them to drive.

I often find myself in the kitchen cooking a big stew or soup. This is what I will eat on the first couple of days of bleeding, when I will not want to cook. I also often get an urge to clean my home just before I begin to bleed. This appears to be very similar to the urge women get before giving birth: preparing the nest. I have talked to many women who share this sudden impulse to clean, clean, clean. This is a very useful biological pull for those of us who do not usually enjoy domestic tasks; it means that you have a clean and tidy space in which to retreat. I also make sure I go shopping to buy plenty of food before my period starts, and get in the firewood, so that I am free to go internally wherever the period wants to take me without having to be pulled out of that precious state by the demands of everyday life.

You may feel a little clumsy just before your period starts. This is due to changes in progesterone levels in your bloodstream which affect the fluidity in your joints, meaning that until you adjust each month to the shifting hormone level, you drop things and stumble. Take care! It is a reminder that it is time to slow down. Be careful when driving and make sure to concentrate harder than usual. If you know you are a bad premenstrual driver, don't drive! Stay home and get your nest ready for a cozy retreat.

Sometimes, just before my period starts, I feel negative and depressed. My thoughts become a little paranoid and life just looks bleak. I have bad dreams and I feel like I am in the dark about everything. My tendency for self-doubt rears its ugly head, and I turn on myself and on my period. Do I really need to go through this mess and cramps and inconvenience and grumpiness and not feeling like going out *every* month? Wouldn't once or twice a year be enough?

This feeling tends to come on when I am waiting for my period to begin. There is a heaviness to my body and I just wish it would start and get on with its thing. At moments like that I feel distant from my body and its processes and impatient with myself and with everyone and everything around me.

My breasts are tender and so is my heart. Everything hurts more: I watch a movie on the television and weep, I cry myself to sleep, I worry about the world. I feel colder than normal, and vulnerable in a raw and aching seemingly neverending way. I have felt this feeling so many times in my life, and yet here I am, warm and dry, with food in my kitchen, clothes on my back, in a better situation for survival than many people on this planet. Yet nonetheless, in the time immediately before I begin to bleed, I am weak and anxious and I want someone, a big cosmic momma, to give me a cuddle and tell me that everything will be all right.

I battle the demons of self-doubt with all the weapons I have gathered over the years. I get on with my work, and tell them, kindly, to please leave me alone. I know that they are just picking on me because I feel vulnerable today. I light a fire to warm the room and my heart. I call a friend. I cook a nourishing, filling meal full of carbohydrates and comfort. I go easy on myself.

This is the moment of darkness before entering the sacred cave. It is an important moment in the initiation of each and every period. Learning to maintain awareness and walk through the premenstrual phase of anxiety, depression and doubt without getting over-attached to any of your personal demons is a preparation for walking into the unknown in every sphere of life and death.

Phase Two : The Major Bleeding and Release Phase

When the first blood comes I look at it and always there is a spark of pleasure, of recognition: ah! there you are again. I get out my cloth pads from their place in the bathroom closet. Sometimes I have a cup of tea to celebrate the return of my blood, and to warm my body. (blood temperature drops as we begin to bleed)

At this point I feel myself going more and more into retreat mode, and I may turn the phone off and actually take some time to be completely alone, depending on my need. The extent of my retreat varies from month to month. Some months are particularly powerful. I remember one month when an image of myself in isolation and silence had persistently crept into my thoughts. When my blood came, the urge for complete silence became very strong. So I turned off the phones, and made an agreement with myself not to turn the television or radio on if I got bored, but just to sit with it. I called a couple of friends and told them that I would be incommunicado for a few days. For five days I spoke to no one, with no external stimulus, no contact with the media in any form.

It was bliss. I wrote, and meditated for long periods of time, finding it unusually easy to go into a strong still place in myself. In the afternoons I went for gentle walks in the park behind my home. I wore no makeup, and barely looked in the mirror.

When I began coming out of this state I looked in the mirror and saw that I looked different; very clear-eyed but rather like someone who is ill, and I realized that illness is partly a retreat into the interior world. I wasn't ill, I felt fine, but my personality wasn't present on my face: I didn't have a face for the outside world. All my energy was focused on something that was happening inside. It took a couple of days for my face to return, for the energy to come back to the surface.

During this time I had several big dreams, and made a leap forward in my understanding of this book and the shape it needed to take. It felt necessary and healing and loving to give myself this time. I felt more centered than I had for a while, and wrote several important letters which represented the completion of two significant relationship problems that had been ongoing in my life. I felt so good during this time it is hard to find words to describe the state. It's not simply that I was happy; it was more than that. I was deeply at home with myself and in touch with the spirit, with a power that is gentle, loving, and vast. I felt that spirit, that energy, suffusing me, filling me up, loving and nurturing me.

But I don't need or want to do such a strong retreat every month. Sometimes it's simply a question of sleeping alone for a night or two and spending some quiet time in meditation during the first couple of days.

While you are bleeding, take some time to notice what this individual period is like and be open to the information offered by any symptoms that arise such as cramps, irregular blood flow, clots, etc. (See Chapter 9 for more on menstrual symptoms.) Follow your dietary instincts very closely. You may not be very hungry for the first day or so, as your body is in cleansing mode. Drink plenty of good water, and nourishing teas. There are some wonderful female tonic herbal teas on the market now that are ideal for drinking while you are bleeding.

Do whatever works for you to help your feelings and thoughts to be cleansed and eliminated along with your blood. If you like to write, you can use your journal as a prod to help your feelings to come out. For some women, painting or sculpture are good ways to release. Do whatever works best for you to allow yourself to let go.

This time can also be very good for creative work that

demands centeredness and focus.

Phase Three : The Emptiness Phase

After the cleansing phase, you will find yourself becoming still inside. Sometimes the emotional cleansing happens more premenstrually, in which case you will feel calm once your bleeding begins. If this is the case, there will still be a noticeable experience of emptiness once the major bleeding is done.

Give yourself open time to just sit. It is wonderful during this phase to sit in nature and just watch the birds and the sky, or look at flowers and trees. You should find yourself spacing out, entering a calm still frame of mind in which nothing much is happening.

I sometimes struggle with the empty time, and start to do things, imagining that nothing is happening internally so I might as well get back to business in the outer world. This rush back into the world has a tendency to backfire and I find that I accomplish little and use up a lot of energy. It's hard to sit still when nothing is coming up to work on; it's hard for me to honor that emptiness even though I know it precedes creativity, inspiration and insight. The empty time is the least dramatic part, and it is important to remind myself to let it happen, and to enjoy it and honor it and not to rush back into the business of life prematurely. If I do that I miss out on the deeply centering gifts at the end of my period.

You will know when you are emptied out. Your blood flow will be less, and you will feel almost bored. Not much is coming up or coming out, psychically or physically. Creative work will probably dry up. Avoid the temptation to end your retreat prematurely and instead, just sit with the empty feeling. Go out into nature and sit on a rock and watch the sunset, or the birds flying overhead and the clouds changing in the sky. Let yourself really slow down. Be nothing.

Phase Four : The Wisdom Phase

At the end of the period, if you have allowed enough time for all the other phases to have their due, you will find yourself in a state of clear knowing. This may be brought to you in the form of a dream, or in a sudden insight during the day. With practice, this wisdom moment becomes a longer period of time, lasting for a day or more, and then begins to operate as a continual background state of mind that infuses everything you experience.

You have to be very open to whatever knowledge each period wants to bring you, in order to successfully notice it and gather it into your conscious awareness. This knowing may refer to the past, the present, or the future, or all three. The knowledge you receive and/or generate within yourself may be entirely personal, it may be interpersonal and to do with other people, or it may be impersonal and dealing with the larger world.

Over time, this practice of honoring the psychological and spiritual rhythm of the period enhances your awareness, so that you become more psychic and more open to spiritual guidance in general. This is a long-term process, so don't expect to turn into a wise and clear being overnight. This is a lifetime work, to gather wisdom every month for the purpose of not only nourishing the present moment, but also of developing yourself into a wise old woman.

Scheduling

If I *have* to do something, some event that was planned months in advance, I have found that I can enlist the help of my cycle. Since I have been honoring my period it has really become my friend. Once I inadvertently planned to run a seminar on the second day of my period. I talked to my body about it the night before, and asked if it would be okay for me to go, as I didn't want to let people down. When I woke up that morning my blood flow was very heavy and I felt rather distraught about having to drive to the venue and then teach, but miraculously, as soon as I left the house I stopped bleeding. After the teaching ended, the bleeding started again. It seemed that the heavy flow in the early morning had been my body going into action to take care of the day's bleeding while I was able to be still and in touch with myself. When I needed to be present for the outside world, the bleeding stopped. I don't recommend abusing the good nature of your body, but it is certainly possible to have a relationship of co-operation and goodwill between the instinctive drive and the conscious will. The instincts have to feel deeply respected, however, otherwise they will rebel against being ignored, and illness or dis-ease of some type will result.

As Wendy Alter says in Chapter 10, when she was working at NASA and aspiring to be an astronaut, her period always came at the most inconvenient time, such as when a crucial traning program had been planned. Nowadays she is paying attention to her cycle and says, "I suppose if it can schedule itself to come at inconvenient times then there's no reason it shouldn't come at convenient times too."

For me, my period is the time when I can least get away with activities that are not in harmony with my deepest self. If I have to go on a planned trip when I have my period, sometimes it is fine, and sometimes not. It seems to depend on how necessary the trip is. If it's a journey that the deeper part of me is really not interested in, then my period will not be accommodating, and will probably be symptomatic, most likely with cramps. If the travel is appropriate and needed, then I can do it with reasonable grace. Because the energy of travel goes against the inward-turning stillness of menstruation, our bodies are particularly sensitive to excessive movement at this time.

Most of us have ignored our instincts and, under social pressure, carried on as normal when we have our period. I suspect that this results in a backlog, so that when we first allow the natural rhythm to emerge, the body-mind needs intensive retreat to mend the damage cause by all the years of ignoring the bleeding. I also think that I may be an extreme case. it is clearly part of my life's work to deeply investigate the mystery and meaning of the menstrual cycle, and this may mean that I have a particularly strong need for retreat at this time. Everyone has to find their own rhythm, their own need for silence, for withdrawal, and for healing.

CLOTH MENSTRUAL PADS

The choices we make at a mundane everyday level are very important. By being mindful about the details of how and where and onto what we bleed, we can achieve an increasingly harmonious relationship between our practical, political, and spiritual selves.

Tampons are convenient but can be a health hazard, causing vaginal and cervical irritation, toxic shock syndrome (which is rare), and by promoting reverse blood-flow back into the uterus, probably contributing to endometriosis (which is becoming more and more common). Not only are tampons a health hazard for the women using them, there are millions of them floating in our oceans and clogging up fishermen's nets. Tampon applicators are particularly problematic as a source of long-term pollution.

Shockingly, tampon manufacturers do not have to disclose the ingredients in their products and we do not know exactly what tampons contain. This is nothing short of a scandal. The lack of regulation means that tampons may contain carcinogens that we don't know about. We do know that because of the paper bleaching process tampons often contain dioxin, one of the most carcinogenic substances known.

Conventional bleached paper disposable pads also contain dioxin. They use up trees and add to the mountains of garbage we plow into the earth. They are also a source of marine pollution, with the plastic backing strips acting as a long-term pollutant like tampon applicators. The pads themselves can take several years to break down in the ocean, and until they do, present a hazard not only chemically, but also to sea life. Birds, fish and turtles die from ingesting paper and plastic in the ocean and on the beaches.

We live in a disposable society and it is very hard not to be a contributor to that. But one thing we can do is to make sure that our periods do not make matters worse, that we reclaim our ability to live in harmony with the planet while we are bleeding. After all, when we see menstruation as a sacred part of life, it is a sad testament that the menstruation of women today contributes to pollution and landfills.

The obvious solution is to go back to using cloth. The idea has echoes of "rags" and pre-war poverty, but in practice I've found that cloth menstrual pads work very well I've been using them since 1989, and I am very happy with them. Using cloth sounds difficult and messy but in practice it's simple and comfortable. The pads are made of soft, cozy, absorbent one hundred percent cotton flannel that fits snugly against the body. They are much more comfortable than paper disposable pads. They don't slide around inside your underwear and you don't need to use a belt or pins. I've not had a single accident. If I do have to use paper pads I have more leakage and spillage than with cloth ones. A friend of mine who bleeds very heavily at night has found that the flannel pads are far superior to throwaways, and last right through the night.

Once a pad has been used, I put it in a small bucket of cold water to soak. When my period is over I use the soaking water to feed my plants, and I put all the pads in the washing machine on a hot wash. If the weather is especially warm, or my blood flow longer or heavier than usual, I may do a wash halfway through. The total time of labor involved is around five minutes. Although there is an initial outlay to purchase cloth pads, they last many years, and over time save you money.

If you are healthy then the pads will not smell while they soak in the bucket, unless the weather is really hot or you leave them for more than two or three days. If your menstrual blood smells bad, it is usually a sign that your body needs cleansing by changing your diet, cutting out all junk food, cutting down on animal products and alcohol, taking appropriate herbs, and if necessary, fasting. Bad smells can also be a sign of infection in the uterus, or some other problem, so go see your doctor and get checked out.

Cloth pads cause no damage to the environment and it's a relief to me to know that my period isn't contributing to marine pollution or landfills. I also enjoy a wonderful feeling of autonomy at not having to rush to the store at the first sight of blood. There is no danger of exposure to carcinogens like dioxin, and no danger of toxic shock syndrome. I am also free from the possibility of contracting any of the nefarious infections caused by tampons and by the lack of circulation that results from the plastic backing of the paper pads. All in all, it's a much better deal. And I like the fact that I get to see my blood; it looks much nicer on a piece of floral flannel than it ever did on a grungy old tampon or a white paper pad.

Using cloth pads is a ritual in and of itself. Getting my pads out marks the beginning of my period. I keep them in a pretty bag in a closet. Soaking them and washing them emphasize for me the cleansing, clearing-up aspect of my period. Giving the water to my plants and to nearby trees reminds me of my connection to nature, to the earth and her cycles, and allows me to feel a bond with the land on which I live and with the trees that I nourish with my blood. Folding the pads up once they are clean, and putting them away when my bleeding has finished, marks the end of the sacred pause in the month that is my moon-time.

For women working outside the home it is often impractical to use cloth pads during the day. You can use them at night and use disposables at work. I really don't like using paper pads any more and so I usually try and think of a way to use my cloth pads whatever the circumstances. One solution that I have used is to carry a plastic lined pouch with me. I quickly rinse out the used pad, pop it in the pouch, and then wash it out properly when I get home. I have also successfully used cloth pads while on vacation: I just take three or four pads with me, and wash them out and hang them to dry in the hotel bathroom.

Since the mid-nineties, non-chlorine bleached paper pads and tampons have become widely available, made by natural product manufacturers and sold in natural food stores. I still don't like tampons, even if they are more ecologically sound, but I do use the new paper pads at times and find them to be a useful alternative to cloth pads for a long day of meetings, or a day of travel. They don't have plastic backing and after disposal have a much shorter breakdown time than conventional pads. It is also much easier now to find cloth pads in whole food stores, as well as getting them by mail order.

If you take these simple steps – finding some time to yourself when you have your period, watching the pattern of your period and investigating your own rhythm, and changing to using environmentally and woman-friendly menstrual products – you will be well on the way to healing yourself of the collective wounds of the feminine. You will enjoy the present moment more, by honoring and actually living your period rather than suppressing it. And you will be creating a more balanced and conscious future, not only for yourself, but for your daughters, your friends, and for women everywhere.

CHAPTER EIGHT

Going Deeper:
Rituals, Practices and Meditations

Once you have established a pattern of taking time out when you bleed, you can begin to go deeper. In this chapter we will explore the sacred aspect of menstruation in more depth by looking at ways to deepen experience through journal-keeping, dreaming, creative projects, rituals, and meditations.

But first, here is a list of questions, followed by a series of exercises, designed to stimulate your menstrual memories and awareness. If you can spend some time answering the questions and doing the exercises, the rest of the information in this chapter will be a richer vein for you to tap into. Menstruation is first and foremost about self-awareness, and the deepening process begins with understanding our preconceptions and social conditioning, and with remembering our own personal experiences. These questions and exercises will help you understand more about how you have been trained to think of your body, and how you can work toward a more enjoyable, loving and conscious relationship with yourself.

QUESTIONS TO ENCOURAGE MENSTRUAL AWARENESS

1. Write down three names for menstruation. Think about them. What do they imply to you about menstruation?

2. Think for a few minutes about what it feels like to have your period (for men, or for girls who have not yet menstruated, imagine what it's like) and write down a few words describing that feeling.

3. Next time you have your period track carefully how you feel about yourself. Make notes about these feelings. Do this for two or three months and then, one day when you are feeling quite steady, look at your notes as if they had been written by someone else, someone living on another planet. What is this person's relationship with her body like?

4. How does it feel to say: "I have my period"? Can you say it anywhere without feeling at all embarrassed?

5. Imagine you are from another planet. What would you think menstruation was if the only information you had to go on was a Tampax commercial?

6. Imagine if men were the ones who menstruated. How do you think they would behave when they had their periods? What would the world be like?

7. Imagine you have special powers and you can tell when a woman has her period. What are the clues that you would use?

8. Just for a minute or two, consider that menstruation is magical. What would be the gift of this magical thing?

EXERCISES

Your First Period

Give yourself some quiet time to focus on your first period. For many women this is a very emotional exercise, as most of us have suppressed parts of this memory because of the pain of what we experienced. Give yourself time to fully remember the thoughts, feelings and body sensations. Ask yourself the following questions: What was your first period like? Where were you when you first noticed you were bleeding? Who did you tell? How did they react? How did you feel about it all?

This is a very effective exercise to do with other women, such as in a women's group. The sharing of painful memories can have a healing effect, allowing you to let go of the past. If you have blocked the memory of your first period, working in a group can help as someone else's recall may stimulate your own. And if you have a positive memory of your first period, sharing that is a gift for other women.

Connecting with Archetypal Symbols

Moon: I've always been fascinated by the moon. As a teenager I remember walking home late one wet night and standing in the light of the full moon and gazing up at her. I became aware of a power that I couldn't name and I spontaneously welcomed the full moon and out of some instinct thanked her. I didn't know then what I was thanking her for, but I did it anyway. A vestigial knowing of her effect on the rhythms of life must have lingered in my psyche.

As a young adult I lived in the countryside in England. I used to work in a village pub three miles from my home and the only way I could get there was on my grandmother's old bicycle. I would cycle back late at night, the dynamo noisily clicking, fairly terrified by one particularly dark and lonely stretch of tree-lined road. If the moon was full I was comforted by her light. It mattered to me if she was full or not; it actually affected my experience of life.

I find that my mental state when I am menstruating is much more diffuse than during the rest of the month. Being on my moon makes me like the moon: dreamy, diffuse, unfocused. From this state a different form of awareness is available: less judgmental and organized than my normal way of being, more open to new information.

Think about how the moon affects you. Start tracking, if you don't already, what phase the moon is in. Notice how your moods and desires change with the moon. Go out to the countryside during the full moon and new moon and notice how different everything is at these times. Let the moon get into your cells more, gaze at it, let its energy in more consciously. Let yourself be inspired and moved and stimulated and taught. Do you notice a change in your mental state at your moon-time? Does this connect in any way to your experience of the moon?

Blood: My goddaughter taught me a great lesson about blood one day when she was three years old and insisted on coming into the bathroom with me. After I got up from the toilet she peered in the bowl and said, "Ooh, look at the blood. It's so beautiful!" Taking her lead, I looked at the blood with a small child's eyes myself, and was amazed to see how truly beautiful it was, this magical rosy red fluid swirling around in the water, looking like life itself.

Most of us are repulsed by our menstrual blood and think of it as dirty. In fact, we are trained to think this way. Do you remember how you thought about menstrual blood when you first began to menstruate? How do you feel about it now? Do you look into the toilet bowl, or do you avert your eyes? What it feels like to see some of your blood staining a sheet or your underwear? Do you feel ashamed of your blood?

Could you paint a picture with it? Daub it around your home as a form of protection and to mark your territory? Use it to feed your plants? Try looking at your blood with the eyes of a small child who is fascinated by life.

Earth: Like many people, I gain a great sense of peace and connectedness from walking in the wilds or simply sitting quietly on the earth or gardening, having my hands deep in the soil. We need this sense of connection to the natural world, to the planet we inhabit. When I've been in the city too long a part of me begins to go crazy and I long for the beach, for the woods, for the feeling of real earth beneath my feet. As a friend of mine once said after living too long in London, "I just want to rip the concrete up off the streets and find the earth beneath it."

Take some time to sit on the earth near where you live. Just sit, and let the energy of the earth come into you. What is it saying? How close do you feel to the earth? Does it seem foreign and more of a concept than a reality? How could you get closer to sensing the earth energies? Try visiting power spots, mountains, lakes, sacred places. When you bleed, go to a private place in nature and let a few drops fall on the ground. Watch what thoughts and images come to you as you do this.

Snake: I used to be terrified of snakes. I couldn't imagine why people would have them as pets. I remember once walking in a park and seeing a man carrying a huge python. I wouldn't go too close, but I stood and stared for a long time; there was intense fascination intermingled with my fear and revulsion.

Then some years later, I was in the rainforest in Central America, studying with a shaman and performing ceremonies. I walked barefoot through the forest one day and felt myself in harmony with the land, and knew that the snake world meant me no harm as long as I was mindful about where I put my feet. Since then I have had only respect for snakes.

The way we relate to snakes has a lot to do with how we relate to our own instincts, to our own deep knowing. Think about times in your life when you have been changed – through illness, emotional trauma, sudden upheaval, through what was known being taken from you – and if you have a negative perception of these changes, try reframing them in the context of the loss of a skin. When you have your period, imagine yourself as a snake, shedding your skin and being renewed for the coming month.

Reimagining Puberty

We don't have any traditional puberty rituals in Western culture that value the onset of menstruation and connect it to the earth and to the power of women. This is an enormous hole in our collective and personal experience, and contributes to the lack of centeredness suffered by so many women. If women were validated and assured of their worth when they went through puberty, they would be far less open to abuse and to self-destructive behaviors like eating disorders.

In the first exercise I suggested remembering your own first period. When you have fully remembered the whole experience, and connected with the archetypal symbols of menstruation in Exercise 2, go back into your memory and give that young girl a different and completely validating experience. Tell her what you wish you had been told.

What would you have liked to have happened when you had your first period? Can you imagine a ritual that would have been a positive experience for you? Does it feel too embarrassing to have so much focus on you at that time?

Imagine living in a world in which there is no embarrassment about having your first period, one in which you feel that you are entering an exciting adulthood and are given every encouragement to develop all your potential strength and wisdom, in ways that feel natural to you as a woman.

KEEPING A MOONTIME JOURNAL

Keeping a journal is a helpful tool for discovering more information about your own rhythm and your own needs and desires within the structure of the monthly cycle. Of course, it is important to stay fluid with the information that comes, because every month is different. And at the same time as every month is different, we each also have our own hallmark ways of menstruating, our own particular brand of PMS, and our own ways of going out of balance and of finding ourselves again. Keeping a journal will help you know yourself better.

To keep a moon-time journal, it's a good idea to make an entry every day with at least the following information: the day of your cycle and the phase of the moon. Then if you have time and feel inclined, you can add in your energy level, body sensations and symptoms, and go further by writing about your dreams, thoughts, and fantasies. Recording your emotional mood and capacity for relating to others is also crucial information that will help you understand how much time out you need, and how to prevent PMS from being an unconscious and destructive force. It is also useful to make note of any synchronicities or unusual occurrences that attract your attention and seem to hold information. Note when you experience yourself as more psychic or aware.

Is there a time in the month when you feel more impersonal and have a harder time dealing with other people? Is there a time when you need cuddles and sympathy from others? Is there a time in the month when you have lots of energy for listening to and taking care of everyone in your circle? Is there a time when you want to take care of the whole world? And is there a time when all you want to do is curl up with a good book or soak in a hot bubble bath and not talk to anybody?

By keeping a daily journal you will always know what day of your cycle you are on and how that relates to the moon's cycle, and you will begin to learn what your own rhythms are. It is important to record impulses even if they are not followed. Here is an example of one day's entry: "January 9th, Day 4, Moon Day 3, in first quarter. Woke up feeling very dreamy; it was hard to concentrate on my work but I persisted."

This exercise is more difficult to do if you are taking hormonal birth control, as your cycle will be distorted as a result. Intrauterine devices affect the menses too. However, it is still helpful to keep a journal and see what is going on.

Keeping a journal can really help you get to know yourself better and then you will be in a better position to honor your body and its cycles. Learn to identify your conditioning and then question it. Notice and record the moments of conflict that arise between your own rhythm and the demands of the world around you. How do you deal with this? Are there creative ways to work around apparent conflicts that leave everyone feeling better, rather than simply pleasing others and feeling neglected yourself, or vice versa? Menstruating with consciousness is a great way to examine the ways you abandon and neglect yourself in favor of others, or in favor of the status quo. Write down what you observe of your process, so that you can work on it month by month.

If you are a meditator, notice what your meditation is like when you are bleeding, and at other times in the cycle. If you are a dreamer, you can use the structure of the menstrual cycle to record how your dreams change during the month.

MENSTRUAL DREAMING

Connie Kaplan, a shamanic dreaming teacher in Los Angeles, teaches that there are four types of beings on the earth who are responsible for dreaming, whose task for the collective involves dreaming for everyone, not just for themselves. These four types of beings are whales, dolphins, male lions, and female humans.[1] We know that whales, dolphins and male lions spend over 95% of their time in either play, lovemaking or sleep. Most women, on the other hand, work very hard and find it difficult to get any time to themselves at all.

Connie Kaplan's information has a truth to it that I find compelling, especially as it fits so clearly into the thesis of this book, which is really just a modernized version of ancient shamanic teachings from all over the world. Women should take time out when they menstruate, and this time is for dreaming. Not just nighttime dreaming, but also daytime dreaming: being free to enter a dreamy state while awake. The period is a profound dreaming time for women. It is the time when we naturally want to spend more time asleep, more time in contemplation, and less time in structured doing. Many indigenous people teach that women should be left alone when they are menstruating, to dream for everyone.

The women's group leader May East grew up in Brazil, and calls her period "hammock time". She spends as much of her period as she can lying in a hammock and entering a dream state. I recommend hammocks as being particularly good places to relax and enter altered states. Being supported by a hammock in the air is a close reminder of the time we spent in the womb, protected and buffered by the amniotic fluid. Hammock time heals us by connecting us to the eternal mother archetype, and allows our bodies to fully relax while gently swaying into a trancelike state. Try falling asleep in a hammock under the shade of a tree on a warm day and let your dreaming take you to new places. Hammock time especially lends itself to the Emptiness Phase of the period, after the emotional discharging is complete and you are feeling at peace.

There is a distinct pattern of dreaming related to the menstrual cycle. According to Patricia Garfield, who has conducted extensive research into women's dreaming, there is clear evidence of a pattern of changing dreams during each cycle. Before and during ovulation, we are more likely to have sexual dreams, social dreams, and dreams with friendly male figures. Just before and during menses the color red often figures in dreams, and male figures may be hostile. According to Garfield's research, women are more prone to have the words "alone" and "gift" in menstrual dreams than at other times in the cycle, which is a fascinating link from the subconscious to the main thesis of this book.[2]

In my experience – from my own dreams and those of my clients and from working with groups of women – I find that during the premenstruum dream content sometimes becomes unpleasant, often including hostile male figures, and exaggerated instances of hurt from the past. These intensified memories come to the surface during the premenstruum to be acknowledged and released. Shadow elements of the personality – aspects of your own nature you have chosen not to identify with and been conditioned not to identify with – will also display themselves during the premenstruum. Try gestalting your dreams at this time, by imagining you are each of the dream figures in turn. This will allow you to begin to reintegrate the disavowed elements of your own nature. Not all dreams need to be gestalted however, and if it doesn't feel right for you, don't do it.

If you habitually dream of violent men, there may be some power locked up in your male side which only comes out in your premenstrual dreams. Try letting your animus out the rest of the month through your creativity and through choosing work that you really love.

Violent dreams sometimes signal unresolved abuse from the past, or ways in the present in which you are experiencing physical or emotional or psychic violence. This abuse may be subtle, but if you are dreaming about it then you are suffering from it, so try and identify its source. Bear in mind that this abuse may be collective, not personal. Women can carry a sense of being abused by the culture in which we live, and not necessarily from their own personal experience. Dreaming that a man hates you and wants to injure you can just as well come from watching too many female-in-jeopardy movies on TV as it does from any actual incidence you may have personally encountered. Carefully monitor what you watch on television just before and during your period. You are more vulnerable at this time; this goes hand-in-hand with being more psychically open and aware. So you may be particularly sensitive to dark energy and negative messages that instill terror and a sense of disempowerment. Try to nourish your psyche by looking at images that are positive and life-enhancing and that make you feel loved and empowered and honored.

Violent dreams can also signal physical imbalance, such as too much heat in the system. If the violent dreams go along with any of the following symptoms, you may need to seek medical advice: fevers, itchy red skin rashes, migraines, irritability, heartburn, indigestion and mouth ulcers. In Chinese medicine, these symptoms indicate excess heat inside the body, and you may want to consult a Chinese medical doctor for help in rebalancing your system using diet, herbs, and acupuncture.

Dream content during the period itself tends to follow the four phases of menstruation described elsewhere in this book, and often precedes the waking experience of each phase. The Preparatory Phase may be signaled by dreams of cleaning, for example, of swimming pools being emptied, or of red wine being poured down drains. The Major Bleeding and Releasing Phase may be immediately preceded by a bad dream, by dreaming of the color red, by an emotional dream. The Emptiness Phase often is ushered in by a night of either no dreams, or peaceful dreams of landscapes, or water, or a sense of quiet pleasure. The Wisdom Phase can begin in the dreamworld as early as Day Two or Three, perhaps by having a dream that sheds light on some crucial matter in your life, and which gradually makes sense to you and filters into your conscious mind fully by the end of your period.

Experiment with your dreaming by asking questions of your dreams before going to sleep and by making a special effort to remember and record them. Sometimes it helps to focus your attention by putting a crystal under your pillow, or by saying a prayer before you go to sleep expressing your desire and intent to listen to the wisdom of your dreams and to remember them.

You can ask your spirit guides to send you dreams on particular subjects, for more information about such matters as the meaning and correct context of a relationship, or what work you should be doing, or what your higher self wants you to focus on right now. If you have a religious practice, you can pray to your preferred deity for help with your dreams. There is a long tradition in all the major religions (sometimes in the esoteric reaches of the religion, but there nonetheless) of people being inspired by and receiving teachings in their dreams.

Keep your journal right next to your bed so that you can write dreams down without having to get up. If you have trouble recalling the dream, try putting yourself in the same body position you were in when you woke up. This often triggers the memory. If you can't remember the whole dream, go back to the part of the dream that you do remember, and relax and let the dream unfold again. If you can't recall the whole thing just write down the part you can get hold of. Often this is where the most energy is in the dream anyway. Notice if there are persistent images that you try to block on waking. Your unconscious wants you to acknowledge something, and it will keep on giving you the image until you register it consciously. You might as well let it happen, because it will speed up your personal development and free you from inner demons.

If you have not yet trained yourself in dream recall, the best way I know to do this is to embark on a rigorous practice of writing down all your dreams, no matter how arbitrary or ridiculous or meaningless they appear to be. If you do this for a year, you will have trained yourself to remember your dreams, and you will then be able to distinguish which dreams are actually worth writing down. If you can, write in the dark, and move your body as little is possible in between waking and recording the dream.

Eventually you will get to the point where you write down just a few dreams every year, and are able work on and absorb the rest of your dreams without needing to commit them to paper. In the beginning though, write down everything. It is really worth doing this, because you will come to understand your own dream life in a way no book or therapist can teach you. They are your dreams, after all. It is of course useful to take your dreams to specialized interpreters sometimes, whether that be a Jungian analyst or a shaman or an intuitive, wise friend. But ultimately, you must take responsibility for your own ability to interpret and get the most from your dream life, because it is as unique an expression of your own beingness as your face and fingerprints.

MOONTIME CREATIVITY

In her work as a menstrual educator, Tamara Slayton encouraged women to use their period as a time of creativity:

> "In one class we make dolls – menstrual dolls, fertility dolls. This is a big part of the work with the younger girls. Art is the access to the imagination. We make little beeswax uteruses; we make greeting cards congratulating each other. During advent we made lanterns, and last time we made golden crowns to honor the Madonna in us – that was really awesome seeing all these women sitting in this room wearing golden crowns – very powerful."

Using the natural creativity of the period to get in touch with yourself through writing and painting can be of great benefit. Often, understanding of deep processes comes more easily through painting and writing than it does through trying to tackle the problem directly. The diffuse state of awareness that comes with menstruation makes this an ideal time for letting go into what Castaneda's Don Juan called the nagual and Australian aborigines call the Dreamtime; the unknown of ourselves where there is wisdom and knowledge. Try writing, painting or drawing about your own experiences of menstruation and of puberty. You may learn unexpected things about yourself when you allow information to come through creative channels. This is also a great way to access information about the future.

SACRED SPACE AND ALTARS

It's a good idea to make a space in your home that is your own sacred place: a room where you can dream, doze, paint, draw, sew, and write. If not a whole room, then at least you can make an altar, a special little shelf or table which acts as a focus for ritual activity and for centering and strengthening of the spirit. Most women have some kind of altar in their home without necessarily ever calling it that: a shelf that holds precious items and photographs of loved ones, a basket of treasures gathered from beaches and woodlands, a plant next to a little statue next to a photo of Grandma. It is just another step in reclaiming our own connection to Spirit to add a candle or two and some sage or incense, perhaps a bowl of water and a little pile of earth or cornmeal. There you have a sacred space, honoring the four elements of fire, earth, air and water, before which to sit and center yourself.

RITUALS

Rituals are valuable for several reasons. As women's ritual leader Hallie Iglehart Austen says in Chapter 12, rituals focus our attention. By focusing our attention, rituals allow information to become available to us that otherwise we might miss.

Rituals also connect us to our atavistic roots, and help us to refind ourselves and experience ourselves in an eternal, non-technological way. Rituals releases hormones and change cell chemistry in ways that are not yet understood by scientific medicine, but which are nonetheless relevant to us.

Our ability to heal ourselves through conscious, life-honoring ritual is an aspect of human power that is well-known in folkloric tradition all over the planet, and has been documented anthropologically, but usually as if it is an oddity we Westerners could not possibly emulate. No one stands to make a profit from people healing themselves and their societies through ritual, so in a culture driven by materialism, no one puts up the money for research to prove it. Instead we are indoctrinated to think that modern pharmaceutical medicines are our only hope for healing, when in many minor illnesses – and sometimes in serious illness too – often a simple prayer, ritual, or meditation, especially when combined with the correct food or herb, can effectively rebalance our systems so that they can heal themselves.

Rituals change and develop to suit the nature of the times. Now is a time when women are beginning to reclaim the power and value of the feminine and along with that, the long-forgotten positive aspects of menstruation. We are all the cocreators of a new way of celebrating being female.

Hallie Iglehart Austen emphasizes the necessity of courage and experimentation. "We can take something from a tradition and make it our own – or maybe take it back to its original meaning. The tradition of the blood of Christ and the wine is I'm sure taken from the menstrual blood."

Experiment with making up your own rituals. The Native American tradition is a good one to borrow from, because it has a strong understanding of ritual and a respect for menstruation. There is great wisdom and inspiration in the European earth-centered folk traditions, now usually practised as Pagan or Wiccan ritual. There are several good books on rituals available to stimulate your own creativity.

Puberty and Remembering Rituals

We can heal the wound of our lack of formal initiation into womanhood by remembering just what it was like when we began to menstruate. Once we have remembered, then we can begin to undo the negativity that was programmed into us. Women's groups have created post-facto puberty rituals in which each member has remembered her menarche, and then the entire group has conducted a positive ceremony as a way to heal the past. These women are also creating first blood rituals for their daughters, out of a desire to give girls a truly positive and affirming experience of becoming a woman.

Moon Rituals

You can make the moon the focus of your ritual. Some Native American women pray to the moon for the healing of irregular cycles: traditionally, they would sit out under the full moon to bring on ovulation, which would then regulate their cycle so that they would bleed on the new moon.

I have found that it is particularly enriching for me to meditate on the moon and make her in some way a part of my menstrual rituals. It pleases some primitive, essential part of my being just to look at the moon each night and register where she is in the sky, how full she is and what planets and stars are close by. Sometimes I wake up in the night and step outside to look at the night sky. This is harder to do if you live in a city, especially in an area with a lot of tall buildings, and you may want to take a trip out to the countryside and find a peaceful spot where you can sit and gaze at the moon for a while.

You can do rituals, either alone or with a group of like-minded women, to celebrate the full or new moon. New moon rituals traditionally are about cleansing, shedding the old, and asking for the new. The new moon is a time to pray for what you want to happen in your life, and is the most powerful time to begin a new project and ask for blessings for it.

The full moon is a time for gathering, dancing, celebration, sexuality, and joy. A great way to enjoy the energy of the full moon is to throw a party and eat good food, drink a little wine, and dance your socks off. Rituals on the full moon focus on gratitude, magic, and asking for help completing projects. If you want to lose weight, and/or cleanse and purify your body, the best time is under a waning moon, the time between full moon and the next new moon. You can ask the moon for help with this, too.

Let yourself tune into the moon and allow the natural energies of the moon to become known to you. Watch how the moon's cycle affects your own mood and energy level, and those around you. There are many anecdotal reports of emergency rooms, delivery wards, dance classes, and pubs being especially full on the full moon. Conversely, parties held on the new moon often fall flat, with low attendance and a feeling of ennui.

If you open up to how the moon affects your mood, and live in harmony with that, your physical and mental health will improve as you will be living closer to a natural rhythm of which we are all a part.

Purification Ritual

In many cultures, purification rituals are performed at the dark of the moon. For example, in the Tibetan Dzog Chen tradition, there is a purification practice every dark of the moon. This involves visualizations and chanting to clean out all your chakras, and a bathing ritual. It's possible that such practices were originally linked to menstruation, because as we have seen, in the absence of artificial light, women menstruate at the new moon.

We can easily incorporate this ancient practice into our menstrual cycle by doing a simple ritual like taking a long bath. I usually have at least one very long bath during my period, in which I am mindful of purifying my body, and of letting go of whatever needs to leave.

It is also good to eat lightly, especially on the first couple of days of bleeding. Drink plenty of water and let your body purify itself.

At the same time as we cleanse ourselves physically, we can pray for help in cleansing emotionally, and we can acknowledge in prayer our intention to be cleansed on all levels by the period.

This purification can be focused on in meditation by asking, "What don't I want to carry around any more?" Think of yourself as a snake shedding its skin, leaving behind the past and being free to move on to the next month.

Invoking Menstrual Goddesses

You can incorporate the invocation and visualization of goddesses associated with the menstrual cycle into your rituals, such as Artemis/Diana (goddess of the moon, the hunt, wild areas and woodlands, and the protector of women), Aphrodite and Isis and Hathor (associated with the full moon, love, sexuality and fertility), Hecate (crone goddess of the dark of the moon), Sekhmet (lion-headed goddess of wisdom, healing and necessary destruction), Kali and the Tibetan dakinis and their skull bowls of blood (destroyers of whatever is phoney or evil, and protectors of the truth).

Simple Personal Rituals

As part of reinforcing your new, positive, female-affirming belief system around your periods, it's a good idea to have a few simple personal rituals. For example, you can wear certain clothes or jewelry when you are menstruating. For years I always wore a pair of Tibetan earrings with a red stone in them, and then they lived on my altar for the rest of the month.

You can make a practice of taking a few minutes when your period comes on to sit in front of your altar and light a candle and some incense or sage, and say a little prayer of gratitude and recognition of the power of your cycle.

Small rituals like these play an important role in reminding us of the sacredness of bleeding. Each time you make a physical act that honors your period, you are saying to your female body, I love and honor you and will take good care of you. Rituals help to counter the ignorance and denial of the power and beauty of menstruation (and, therefore, of being a woman) that is all around us in our culture.

Blood Rituals

Bleeding onto the Earth: Making the Sacred Connection

When I was first introduced to the idea of bleeding onto the earth by a friend of mine I thought it sounded a little silly, a little pretentious. But I started doing it tentatively, and began to feel a flicker of connection to something very old. One of the problems I had was figuring out how to do it. Native American women traditionally bled onto moss, while sitting on the earthen floor of the moon-lodge. Where was I supposed to sit and bleed? Even if I went and found a nice piece of earth to sit on, I didn't want to stay there for the whole time. Then I started using cloth pads to absorb my blood and soaking them in water before I washed them. I realized that I could pour the soaking water onto the earth. So now that's what I do. The water is a beautiful red, and I pour it onto the ground around plants, and the act of doing this fills me with a feeling of connection, of rightness, of being at peace with something that is often neglected in modern life. These simple acts of value, simple knowledge, are like chopping wood, rocking a baby, baking bread, or drinking from a fast-flowing mountain stream. Bleeding on the earth is one of those acts of being a human being that is of eternal value, part of the steady round of life and death. The cells that die in my body, that are carried in the menstrual blood, are food for the earth. What dies gives birth. What dies feeds those who live and will live.

If I ignore my blood, I get distanced from this knowledge. I fear and dislike my blood, for without the knowledge that it too is food, that it too is a gift I bear, then I see it as purely loss. A waste of blood, a waste of time, a baby that wasn't conceived. Whether I desire pregnancy or not, my blood is always a gift. And it is a gift in a literal sense, as well as a psychic gift to myself. It is a gift from my body back to the earth: the mother that has fed and nurtured me every day of my life.

Women's blood is not waste. It is fertilizer for the earth. This was known by all the earth-centered peoples, by those who revered the Goddess and who recognized the female and her body as the conduit through which life comes, and therefore sacred. This life comes not only in the form of offspring, but also in the form of precious blood, given every month to feed the earth, the plants and insects, and all the beings of the planet. This is another aspect of the miraculous interplay between woman and life. We waste this precious resource, just as we waste the rich placenta after birth, because we fail to recognize the value of the female. We look on this blood, full of iron and other minerals, and all we see is waste matter and so we pour it into our sewage systems, instead of doing the obvious and pouring it onto the earth.

This is simple knowledge. You don't have to study hard, you don't have to read any books at all, you don't take any exams or pick up any diplomas. No one will pat you on the back and say how clever you are or how hard you have worked. The reward is purely internal: in the feeling of being in harmony with something so essential to human life, something that we have taken for granted for the last few hundred years.

One of the most effective ways to ground yourself when you move house is to shed your menstrual blood upon the land of your new home. Then your cells are literally on the land, the land is fed and recognized by you, and you have created a psychic and cellular link with the earth. This has a powerful effect on your relationship with your home territory. It is like an animal making its mark, and it is also an act of love: to give a part of oneself to the land creates a two-way relationship, rather than the one-way attitude that we normally have toward the land that we live upon. As Hallie Iglehart Austen recommends in Chapter 12, you can do this even if you live in town. Take an hour or so to visit a park, or sit in your back garden, and let a few drops of your blood embrace the ground. Bleed at the foot of a tree that you particularly like, and watch your relationship with that tree develop. You will notice the tree in a new way, and feel a bond that is not often experienced by people who do not live close to nature.

The earth emits a pulse to which we are all attuned. This pulse regulates our heartbeat and the cycles within our bodies, from the steady round of the blood pulsing through the veins to the monthly emission of blood from the menstruating woman. This pulse emanating from the earth is very, very subtle. Few people can actually feel it, but that does not mean that it isn't there.

The indigenous inhabitants of the Amazon rainforest recognize the existence of this pulse, and they listen for it when they go in search of the climbing vine that is one of the chief constituents in their sacred tea: ayahuasca. "By listening for a drumbeat that emanates from the vines on the astral plane, talented feitores can locate those sites in the rainforest where the greatest concentration of vines will be found." [3]

Mountains are strong places to feel the pulse. The sacred mountains of the world send out this sound, this rhythm, such as Uluru (Ayers Rock) in Australia and Mount Shasta in California. Lakes and rivers are also good places to tune into the energy of the earth, especially large lakes such as Lake Tahoe and Lake Baikal.

Listening to this pulse comes most easily to the woman in her bleeding time. Then she is open to the mystery of the pulse and the wisdom it contains. When you are in the pulse and can feel it, then you are in the hands of the Goddess, of the great mysterious force from the inside of the planet. Your body is healed and strengthened by the direct contact with and knowledge of this pulse. This is what women are listening to in their bodies – consciously or not – when they sit still during menstruation, when they sit still and they bleed upon the land. This is the deeper meaning behind sitting on the land and bleeding directly onto it.

Blood Vision Ritual

The red dot that Hindu women paint on the third eye is a symbol of the menstrual blood. Originally women would have painted their third eye with their literal blood, and the magic of the blood opened the sixth chakra (the energy center associated with spiritual and psychic vision). The visionary aspect of menstruation is clearly invoked by this practice. The blood carries in it the cells of the body, and therefore it contains the knowledge of the DNA. The genetic code, the lineage, is contained within the bloodstream. Every cell in the body is a microcosm of the whole. By painting the third eye with our blood we open ourselves to the knowledge hidden in the genetic code. This knowledge includes deep ancestral awareness and can bring understanding of our own family patterns and also of the human family.

We all have within us the knowledge of every generation of human beings that has ever lived. Locked into that coding is a mass of information gathered throughout history. At times the information sleeps; at times it wants to come alive again. We are living at a time when the knowledge of the earth, of the female, is surging back into the collective awareness, and through our blood we can tap into it. Next time you bleed, try connecting consciously with your blood. Try painting a gentle red dot on your forehead, and see what knowledge from the earth and from our ancestors flows into your consciousness. Paint a dot on your third eye before going to sleep to enhance your dreaming.

Blood Creativity Ritual

Experiment with using your blood in art, as a paint. Try painting on rocks and stones as well as on paper or fabric. Make a ritual painting of yourself menstruating, either using your blood or red paint. In this way you combine honoring your blood and reclaiming it as a sacred fluid with creativity and ritual. Let yourself gently go into the altered state that exists around menstrual blood. Let your blood transform you.

MENSTRUAL MEDITATIONS

First, a word on bellies. In order to meditate properly you have to breathe deeply and in the process, let your belly fully relax. For many people, deep abdominal breathing is difficult because they are habitually tense in the belly region. And if we can't relax our bellies fully then we can get menstrual problems from tension and tightness which impede smooth blood and energy flow in the lower abdomen.

Letting the belly go soft can be a challenge in today's culture. The violence of our times and of the images we see daily on television can make us tense up in the belly region to protect ourselves. This is an instinctive reaction, but perhaps more damaging to women is the current notion that women shouldn't have bellies at all.

Our current cultural preference in the Western world for flat and androgynous teenage bellies has several causes. One is our denial of the power of the womb. In cultures where the feminine is more respected and honored, such as India for example, the roundness of women is considered beautiful, and in fact women strive for curves and flesh.

When we take back the reality of being women and the power contained within the generative cycles of our beings, then the belly comes back into its own as the home of the womb and ovaries. The belly is also of course the home of the digestive process, which is also a part of life that we culturally ignore. We tend to eat food fast and without ceremony, without saying thank you or grace, without allowing restful time for digestion to lovingly and fully take place. Instead we jump up the minute we have eaten so we can get back to Doing Things.

Fear of the aging process and overidentification with youth also promotes a denial of the belly. Men and women don't develop bellies until maturity, and usually not until after pregnancy for women and middle-age in men. Thus the belly is a signal that youth is gone forever, and in a culture that venerates youth above sagacity, there is little to be gained in the eyes of one's peers from having a belly. I don't say this in order to support laziness and lack of fitness. Having healthy stomach muscles and a generally trim and fit physique is always to be lauded, but it is natural for women to have more rounded stomachs than men; look at old paintings or photographs of women from other cultures. It is a modern phenomenon to expect women to have flat stomachs, just as it is a modern phenomenon to rush away from the table once you have eaten; or worse, to eat standing up and on the run. This denial of the reality of the belly also ties in with pretending that nothing is happening when you have your period.

So, to meditate, you need to fully relax and breathe deep into your belly, and I know of no better introduction and encouragement for this than the following exercise:

Soft Belly

I learned a meditation called "Soft Belly" from Stephen Levine at a lecture he gave some years ago. It was very effective, and I went round for days afterwards incanting Soft Belly, Soft Belly, gently under my breath and being aware of the many subtle ways I would hold and tense my belly as I went through my day. Soft Belly, Soft Belly. That's all it is really: just focus on your belly and allow it to soften. You may want to go into the tension first: feel how tense it can get, make it really tense and experience that and then say softly to yourself "Soft Belly" and allow the tension to float away, and feel the release and the happiness, the peace and easiness of having a soft non-judgmental happy little belly full of love and compassion and tenderness for the world and everything around you.

Let go into that softness and allow it to spread all over your body and feel the luscious loveliness of your whole being and the juicy delicious femaleness of having a soft and pliable, a warm and comforting belly. A place for babies to grow, a place for feelings to develop, for ideas to gestate, for food to be digested and fully absorbed, a place for all your feelings to be worked on and out and through, a place for cozy late night suppers and happy active early morning breakfasts, a place for comfort, for solitude, for lying on the earth feeling the hot sun on your warm back as your soft and tender loving belly caresses your mother, the earth.

Relax more deeply into your belly now. Feel the goddess within you, she loves your round and full belly, she loves the femaleness of you, the fecund weightiness of that full soft belly. Let it go even more. Softly, softly, your belly is rounding out, letting go, and you are coming home, more and more at home with yourself, as you release the images of a flat and masculine teenage non-belly, for now you are a woman who has given or who can give birth to another being, and to do that you need a belly. So let your belly be, be proud of it, wear it in the world along with your big heart and your shiny eyes, wear your round soft tender loving belly out into the world and soften all around you with the power of your soft and tender loving belly. And when a child is crying pull him onto your lap and let him sit on your belly, and when your inner child is crying put your hands on your belly and rub it softly saying, it's OK, I'm here, and here is our soft and tender, loving belly, the center of our being, the home of our womb, the center of gravity, the deepest place within, and nurture that belly space, for within it is the treasure trove of your creativity, and your gift for the world.

Meditation on Change

The menstrual cycle is an alchemical process, during which every women who bleeds goes through a transformation inside herself. Every month is an opportunity for change and development.

You can become a conscious cocreator in the alchemical process of your menstrual cycle by taking some time during your period to consciously meditate on your life and on ways in which you would like to change. The best time to do this meditation is toward the end of your period, after the cleansing phase, when you are open and empty.

Let your mind be open and ask for information about change in the coming month, or whatever time period you are focused on. Let images arise and watch them. It takes practice to be able to do this kind of imagination work, but everyone can do it. If images are not the most natural way for you – if you are not predominately visual – then allow sounds, words, body feelings, smells to arise. Information will come. Just sit still for a while, relax fully, and ask the questions: "What information would be useful for me to have right now, for the coming time?" "In what ways would it be good for me to change, to grow and develop over the next month?" If nothing comes to you in the session, watch your dreams that night. Sometimes the conscious mind blocks information from the unconscious while we are awake, but when you have given the permission, and the trigger, the information will come during your sleep.

*   *   *   *

To menstruate means to live through a monthly cyclical transmutation in which the past is shed and the new is embraced. Experiencing this transformation through conscious ritual and meditation awakens us to our connection with the cycles taking place all around us, and to our relationship with all life.

CHAPTER NINE

Natural Remedies for Menstrual Symptoms

This book has focused on how our attitudes and belief systems affect our menstrual well-being and our sense of ourselves as powerful women. While attitudes are an important part of health and lead to beneficial behavioral changes, sometimes we need to use medicines to help our bodies realign.

Human beings have always used plants and special exercises to balance their bodies and create healing. The innate wisdom of our bodies and the gifts of the plant world are our primary healing tools. Taking care of ourselves and really loving ourselves as women also means knowing what food to eat, what herbs to take, and how to move our bodies to generate healing.

In this chapter, I describe ways to heal menstrual symptoms using gentle, time-honored methods such as yoga, herbs and foods. There are many resources at our disposal that are nontoxic and that refresh and rejuvenate our cells, creating less symptomatic periods and premenstrual experiences, and helping our overall health.

Since the 1970's there has been a remarkable revival of woman-oriented healing lore, which has coincided with the general upswelling of information about the relationship between our health and the natural world. Practitioners working in the natural healing fields have married old wisdom with contemporary needs and have developed some new methods to deal with menstrual symptoms that, when used mindfully, can augment the attitudinal and behavioral changes that I have discussed in the rest of this book.

The first part of this chapter describes different healing methods and how they can be specifically used for menstrual health. The second part lists menstrual symptoms, and suggests the most effective and natural ways to alleviate them.

HEALING METHODS

Food

Food is often the best medicine. It is relatively cheap and readily available. Our bodies recognize food and can use it to heal without any strain on the system. Our digestive systems know how to metabolize food and make the most of it. Ideally, we should always eat what our bodies want to eat. Unfortunately, the stress of modern life, abuse of dieting, and so-called scientific ideas about food (often influenced by commerce) have tended to separate us from our food instincts and we often follow food fads in the mistaken belief that it will be good for us.

The following information is given with the caution that if eating a recommended food feels wrong for you – especially if you hate the taste – then don't eat it. The most important element here is to learn to listen to your body. Unfamiliar food should be tried at least once, unless you have a really strong instinct that it will be bad for you, because if we were raised on a diet of limited variety our body-mind becomes limited in terms of what foods it thinks are acceptable.

If your body is carrying a high load of toxicity, your ability to discern what food you need will be severely impaired. So what you need to do first is to find a good naturopathic doctor who can take you through a cleansing program. When your body is detoxified you will be in a far better position to follow your food cravings and desires. The same also holds true if you have addictions to food or any other substance. Once your body is clear of the addictive substance and no longer confused by trying to maintain balance amidst an overload of sugar or drugs or nicotine or whatever, you will be reunited with the food instinct you had as a baby.

In the week before your period begins, try and avoid salty foods which may cause water retention, and fatty foods and alcohol which tend to heat up the liver function and exacerbate PMS. In Chinese medicine the liver is considered responsible for hormone regulation, and it is usually liver imbalance that creates premenstrual depression and irritability. Alcohol, and foods which can irritate the liver, such as caffeine and spicy foods, may make PMS worse.

If you feel sluggish and your digestion slows down during this week, try taking fresh lemon juice in hot water first thing in the morning, to stimulate the cleansing processes of the liver. Grapefruit will also do this.

It is quite natural and in keeping with your bodily needs to eat a little more during this week, and to crave carbohydrates. Just try and eat whole grains, be very moderate in your intake of sugars and refined foods, and stay off junk foods completely. If you want to eat chocolate, which can be balancing at this time, eat a small amount of very good quality chocolate. Be aware that sugar robs the body of B complex vitamins, so eating sugar premenstrually will exacerbate any B deficiency that you have.

During the period itself, while you are actually bleeding, it is best to eat lightly as your body is in a cleansing phase. But if the weather is cold or you just feel hungry, eat what your body needs. It is important to eat warm and cooked foods during your period, even in summer. Stay away from iced foods and cold-energy foods such as cucumber and melon, which when eaten during menses deplete the spleen function (which governs the blood in Chinese medicine) and may induce menstrual cramps. Foods which are nourishing to the spleen and therefore good during your period include easily digestible grains such as millet and sticky rice (very well-cooked rice), and naturally sweet foods such as root vegetables (well-cooked), stewed fruit, sweet potatoes, dates and honey. Again, be cautious with sweet foods at this time, and only eat what feels right and balancing for you. Having a little sweetness in a meal aids digestion and assimilation, which is why we often crave something sweet at the end of the meal, but too much is unbalancing, and most modern desserts are too large and too sugary. Ice cream is particularly bad during the period, because it is too cold, too sweet, and too rich in fats. Save it for a very hot day in the middle of your cycle, and look on it as a rare treat.

Toward the end of the period, it's a good idea to eat some

blood-nourishing foods rich in iron, such as lamb (especially lamb's liver, if you can find meat raised without hormones and antibiotics), beets, blackstrap molasses, eggs, dried fruit, and green leafy vegetables.

Supplements

Supplements are popular these days, and can be helpful. However, I would like to sound a note of caution about their use. Vitamin and mineral supplements are powerful, can be impure, have the potential to unbalance your body, and should be used only when other more gentle methods have proved to be insufficient, or if you have been medically diagnosed with a lack of a specific vitamin or mineral.

There is a tendency at the moment, among both healthcare professionals and the pseudo-scientific media such as women's magazine articles, to advocate large doses of vitamins and minerals without making a clear diagnosis or establishing a clear treatment protocol. I don't think that taking megadoses of these substances is a good idea in the long-term. They are a crude attempt to make up for the lack of nutrition in our food caused by modern farming methods and pollution. If you eat locally-grown organic produce, drink filtered water, moderate your stress level through relaxation and yoga, and use natural anti-oxidants such as green tea and citrus fruits, you can stay healthy without using supplements.

That said, there are some supplements that can be very useful in treating menstrually-related symptoms. Just take them with care, stop taking them when your body is back in balance, and substitute foods rich in these substances instead. Under the list of symptoms at the end of this chapter you will find reference to which supplements can help which menstrual complaints.

Herbs

For millenia, women have used herbs to alleviate their menstrual symptoms and to balance their hormones. This knowledge has been maintained and passed down through the generations despite attempts by patriarchal religious groups and physicians to disempower women.

In recent years, herbalism has been enjoying a renaissance as we come to realize that using the whole plant can have advantages over using isolated ingredients in powerful pharmaceutical drugs which have damaging side-effects. And what we are discovering is that often, and especially in the case of non-life-threatening conditions, herbs can be the most effective and the safest healing method at our disposal.

Herbal plants are all around us, and are part of the organic wholeness of the planet. Animals know what herbs to eat when they get sick, and so did we in more instinctual times. While it may feel like a daunting prospect to reconnect with those atrophied healing instincts and live in a state of harmony and healing with our natural surroundings, we can begin the journey. We can avail ourselves of the knowledge passed on to us by past and present herbalists, many of whom were and are women.

The following are a few of the most often-used and effective herbs for rebalancing and maintaining menstrual health. They are all nontoxic in sensible doses, and simple to take. All the herbs mentioned in this section are easily obtainable, if not from your local wholefood store, then from herbal mail-order catalogs. Some of these mail-order catalogs are specifically for women and carry combinations of herbs already made up for female symptoms, such as period pains or PMS. For more information on herbs for women, I highly recommend the work of Amanda McQuade Crawford (see bibliography).

Chamomile Chamomile is a splendid and gentle relaxant and tranquilizer that will also help you sleep. Chamomile is very good for premenstrual days and nights. Make tea using loose chamomile flowers. If you use tea-bags, which are wonderfully convenient of course, make sure they are good quality and not too old; don't use a moldy old bag that's been lying around your kitchen cabinet for two years.

Cramp Bark (Viburnum opulus) Cramp bark is a muscle relaxant and – surprise, surprise – is great for cramps. The part used is the stem bark of the guelder rose, also known as the highbush cranberry or snowball tree. Cramp bark is non-toxic, although you must not eat the fresh berries from the plant, which are toxic. Cramp bark is an excellent remedy because it relieves pain quickly but does not make you drowsy like some other muscle relaxants. Best taken in tincture form; one teaspoon (5 ml) three times a day. Or you can make tea and drink a cup three times per day, or add the tea to your bath, or blend it with a linament and rub it on your lower abdomen.

Chasteberry (Vitex agnus-castus) Chasteberry normalizes female hormones, and is great for PMS, irregularity of the cycle, and period pains. It is often used in combination with Dong Quai and Black Cohosh to balance hormones. Best taken under the supervision of an herbalist, as are the other powerful women's herbs such as Black Cohosh (Cimicifuga racemosa), Blue Cohosh (Caulophyllum thalictroides) and Dong Quai (Angelica sinensis).

Ginger Ginger is one of the best anti-nausea remedies, so it is useful if you suffer from nausea around the beginning of your period. Drink ginger ale, or better still, make hot ginger tea by chopping a few slices of fresh ginger root and pouring a cup of boiling water on it and letting it steep for five minutes. Taken this way, ginger is very warming, and so it is good if you tend to feel chilly around the onset of bleeding, and if you have cold-type dysmenorrhea (i.e. period pains made better by the application of heat).

Nettles Nettles are a wonderful remedy for women, rich in iron and other nutrients, and symbolically representative of the ability to draw clear boundaries and protect oneself. In the spring, a cup of freshly-brewed nettle tea taken daily for a month will cleanse your liver and kidneys and nourish your blood. This is an old European practice for cleansing the system after the less active winter in which one ate more fatty foods to keep away the cold. It is a great spring-clean for your body, ensures that you will have plenty of vibrant energy for the active summer months, and energizes your entire reproductive system. It's best if you can pick fresh nettles yourself, but if you live in town or in a part of the world where nettles don't grow, you will find that whole food stores and herbalists will have freshly dried nettles by early April.

Nettles can be taken at any time of the year as a general fortifier and specifically for anemia. Too high a dosage can result in an internal feeling of mild irritation; I have found this happens if you let the tea steep for too long in the pot. Five minutes is just right. Use a teaspoonful of the herb for every cup of tea required. If you want to drink a cup three times a day, as for the spring cleanse, for example, in the morning put two or three teaspoonfuls of the dried herb in a medium-sized teapot and cover with just-boiled water. Strain after five minutes and drink a cup there and then and save the remaining two cups to drink cold during the day. Don't keep the decoction in the fridge though, and make a fresh batch every morning. You can also combine the nettles with raspberry leaves, making your cleanse even more female-specific, and tonifying your womb at the same time.

Raspberry leaves Raspberry leaves tonify the womb, and prepare it for pregnancy and childbirth. The tea has a nourishing effect on the uterus and helps stimulate normal function, so it is good for young girls beginning to menstruate as well as for women in general. If you are recovering from a miscarriage or abortion, drinking raspberry leaf tea daily or taking capsules will help your womb to heal and your cycle to reestablish itself.

Essential Oils

Essential oils are derived from plants and have been popular in Europe, especially in France, for centuries. They have enjoyed a revival in recent years and are now widely available at whole-food stores. The therapeutic use of essential oils is called aromatherapy.

Essential oils are best used externally, and I would not recommend ever taking an essential oil internally unless you are under the supervision of an experienced professional aromatherapist who has had medical training. Essential oils taken internally can be highly toxic and can cause lasting organ damage. Care must also be taken when using oils externally, as excessive doses can cause allergic and irritation reactions. If in doubt, don't use more than ten drops of a single essence in a bath, and two drops in an inhalation bowl of hot water.

Dissolved in hot water, the drops can be inhaled, rapidly entering the blood supply through the tissues of the nose. And when used in baths, massage oils and linaments, the oils enter the tissues through the skin, and quickly circulate to the needed areas of the body. A good way to put oils into bathwater is to dissolve a few drops of the oil in a small glass of milk (not skim/non-fat). The oils bond with the fat in the milk and disperse, so in the bath you get a suspension of diluted oils, rather than big globs that won't dissolve properly in the bathwater.

Here is a list of essential oils that help with menstrually-related complaints and would be a useful part of the home medicine cabinet.

Basil is the best aromatic nerve tonic. It is useful for PMS when you feel anxious, depressed or mentally wrung out.

Clary sage is a pick-me-up. It stimulates liver function and makes you feel instantly more cheerful. It is an excellent remedy for premenstrual depression. Clary sage acts as a tonic for the uterus and as a euphoric for the mind. It can be used for cold-type dysmenorrhea and amenorrhea.

Chamomile oil, like the tea, is calming, soothing, and analgesic. It can be used for all menstrual disturbances, especially when there is anxiety along with the physical difficulty.

Geranium balances hormones and helps regulate the cycle, and smells great. You can combine it with rose oil for a wonderful bath.

Juniper is a diuretic, a nerve tonic and a sedative. Juniper stimulates the circulation, so it is good for painful periods when you feel congested, mentally as well as physically. Hence it can also be good for the kind of PMS when you chase the same old negative thoughts around and around your head. Juniper gets things moving, whether it be stuck fluids (water retention), stuck blood (delayed, staccato, and/or painful, spasmy bleeding), or stuck thought-patterns.

Lavender harmonizes and balances and is great as a calming tranquilizer after a hectic day. Lavender is very good for generating peace of mind premenstrually, and for aiding relaxation during the period itself. Lavender balances the nervous system and is very low in toxicity but nonetheless, don't overuse if you have heavy periods because it can increase bleeding. Because of this, it is a good remedy for scanty periods or amenorrhea. Lavender also protects and clears energy, so it's very handy to take when you travel to clear the energy in a hotel room, for example, and to inhale if you feel anxious or stressed out, psychically invaded, or emotionally overwhelmed.

Marjoram warms and relieves spasm and so it is good for cold-type dysmenorrhea. Marjoram is particularly useful for physical and mental conditions stemming from grief.

Melissa (lemon balm) acts as a tonic to the uterus. It calms spasms, making it useful for period pain. It also helps regulate the cycle and it increases fertility. Melissa is soothing and relaxing, and works to remove tensions and blocks. It is good with lavender when work pressures overwhelm your peace of mind.

Rose is the female oil par excellence and makes you feel more feminine, balancing hormones and relaxing and healing the tender heart. If life feels bruising and mean, take a rose bath and relax into the sheer goodness of the essence of rose. Rose helps counterbalance feelings of self-loathing during the premenstrual phase or during bleeding, and brings in a sense of deep self-love and enjoyment of the sensuality of being female. Rose also acts as a gentle emmenagogue (stimulates bleeding), cleansing the womb of impurities and regulating the menstrual function. It is the least toxic of all the essential oils.

Rosemary is the remedy for headaches. It is a nerve stimulant and clears the mind. Use it for premenstrual headaches and menstrually-related migraine. Put a couple of drops in a bowl of hot water and with a towel over your head, breathe deep. If your head already feels hot, don't do this. Instead, either inhale directly from the bottle, rub a drop of the oil diluted in almond oil onto your temples, or spray the room with a few drops shaken rapidly into a spray bottle full of water.

Movement

Often menstrual discomfort is the result of stuck pelvic energy arising from one or more causes: blocked sexuality, abortion and miscarriage, sexual abuse or trauma, fear of living from the instinctual gut level, or inability to ground properly. Movement can do wonders for blocked energy and reflect back on our state of mind, helping us to feel more free while at the same time easing physical symptoms and allowing blood and energy to flow correctly.

Taking a regular yoga class can be beneficial. Some poses in particular can be used as first aid for cramps, and if done during the month will act as a preventative by stimulating blood supply to the lower back and pelvis. Try the Cobra pose, in which you lie on your stomach and then lift your upper torso and head off the floor, supported by your arms, hands flat to the floor and under your shoulders. This pose bends the small of the back and increases blood supply in and out of the pelvic region. Stretches to open the groin and the hips are also helpful.

Belly dancing is an excellent form of movement for loosening up the lower abdomen and getting your energy focus lower down in the body. Most of the exercises in belly dancing promote blood flow to the belly and pelvis. It is also a very sensual way to move and connects us into an old and pro-feminine experience of being female. The movements are natural, sexual and healing.

Another way to move your pelvic energy is a movement I call

the butt wiggle. Stand with your legs shoulder-width apart, bend your knees and stick your bottom out and just shake from the base of your spine, letting your legs hang freely out of the pelvic bowl. You will feel delicious sensations moving up your spine and down your legs, and you will release all the tension stored by standing upright for too long. Let yourself feel the animal in your skin, and hoop and holler at the same time if it feels right to do so. Jumping slightly off the ground with alternate legs can help this energy movement to really flow.

And of course, there is sex. Orgasms can relieve menstrual cramps and certainly promote blood flow to the genitals and the entire pelvic region, as well as stimulating circulation all over the body.

Heat and Water Therapy

Heat and water are old standbys of naturopathic medicine and can be wonderful, simple, effective remedies for many menstrual complaints.

Most dysmenorrhea is better for heat, so try taking a warm bath or using a hot water bottle or an electric pad. I prefer hot water bottles to heat pads as I try and keep the amount of external electricity around my body to a minimum. Hot baths can be soothing and relaxing, especially if you add some essential oils to the water. Don't sit in a too hot bath for too long as it can be enervating. If you find your cramps get worse from heat, stop the application of it, and make sure you get a check-up in case you have a pelvic infection or endometriosis.

A cold water sitz (hip-level) bath for five minutes can help stop excessive bleeding. Alternating cold and hot baths have been used to treat pelvic infection, stimulating blood flow to the area.

For menstrually-related migraines, try bringing the excessive heat in the head down the body by applying cold packs to the temples and back of the neck, and at the same time applying heat to the feet. This works if you have the kind of migraines characterized by a hot head and cold feet.

Castor Oil Packs

For congestion, when your period won't start and you know it's ready but you are blocked for some reason, try a castor oil pack. Castor oil is a purgative and a major detoxifier, and using the packs has been shown to not only stimulate circulation and move the blood, but also to raise the amount of white blood cells in the area to which the pack is applied, so they are good for infections as well.

You need pure castor oil and a pure cotton or wool pack. These are both available from wholefood stores and come with instructions for use. Soak the pad in castor oil and place it on your abdomen with a hot water bottle or heat pad on top. Use a layer of thin plastic between the pad and the heat source, and put a towel over the whole thing to help keep the heat in. Leave this on your belly for twenty to thirty minutes, to allow the heat to help the castor oil to penetrate through your skin.

Don't use a castor oil pack too often, because your body should not be forced to detoxify faster than it can tolerate, and if you use the pack too much you will bleed more and have too frequent periods as your body uses your menses as a way to detox the lower abdomen. Once a week is usually about right. Castor oil packs are good for endometrial build-up which sometimes occurs in perimenopausal and menopausal women, as the castor oil stimulates the womb to fully clean out.

Alcohol

Alcohol tends to heat the liver, and is generally contraindicated for women with PMS. However, alcohol can act a relaxant if you feel tense after a hard day, and if you drink a small amount of good quality red wine or good quality beer (one small glass at the most) with dinner, alcohol in moderation can be helpful for menstrually-related tension. Red wine is also an anti-oxidant and a digestive aid. The more naturally made, preservative-free and well-aged the wine, the better.

Many alcoholic drinks produced today are unhealthy because

of the preservatives and chemicals added to the manufacturing process. Just follow your best judgment, and remember: moderation in all things. If there is alcoholism in your family you may be susceptible too, so find other ways to relax and enjoy yourself. Binge drinking and regular drinking of more than one glass every now and then are harmful to the female body and will exacerbate any menstrual disturbance.

Breath Therapy

If your period feels stuck, if you have pain, if you feel uncomfortable, breathing into your belly, sacrum and womb can release tension and reduce pain and discomfort. Sit or lie somewhere peaceful, light a candle and some incense, and allow yourself to sink your attention down into your lower abdomen. Breathe deeply, focusing the breath on different areas, and experiencing the sensations that come. Allow any tears or fears to arise and leave. Let yourself be healed by the power of your own breath. Ask your spirit guides/God/favorite deity for help and healing. Thank them for the joys and teachings of the previous month, and ask for whatever you need for the coming month, for example, strength, courage, money or love. Your cramps will ease up as you relax into the power of your spiritual connection through the vehicle of conscious breathing.

Energy Clearing

You can do a lot by yourself to maintain a clear energy field. There are several techniques which can help bring us back to balance and these are especially useful after a trying day at work, after dealing with difficult people, after a fight, after a shock, after being with someone who has drained your energy, or after being in the city surrounded by exhaust fumes.

Smudge Smudging is a Native American way of cleansing and purifying the energy field, by burning dried herbs and standing in the smoke and waving it around your body. Smudge itself is the name given to the herbs which you burn and whose smoke you use to cleanse negative energy and also to bring in new energy. Use sage to purify, cedar to bring in wisdom, lavender to bring in beauty, and copal to open the third eye and encourage visions. Put the dried herbs in an abalone shell and light with a match. These days, smudge sticks are available from wholefood stores and bookstores. Incense also performs the same functions, but I have found that nothing beats sage for its calming and cleansing and centering properties.

Visualization If you don't have any smudge, or are not in a situation where using it is appropriate, you can visualize your aura being cleansed. Imagine golden light coming down and washing away any dark or cloudy energy from around your body. Or ask the earth to absorb any negativity in your field, and imagine that cloudiness being taken into the earth and transformed. Make up your own visualizations that are appropriate to the situation.

SYMPTOMS AND RELATED TREATMENTS

Premenstrual Syndrome

Symptoms: anger, irritability, depression, water retention, premenstrual acne.

Inner work Are you angry or frustrated about something in your life that needs to change? Are you letting someone invade your boundaries in an unhealthy way? Are you unhappy about a situation in your life but in denial about it the rest of the month? Are you allowing your female sensitivity enough space, or are you colluding with others or with society to desensitize yourself?

It is a mistake to think that premenstrual anger or irritability is always unjustified or pathological. Often precisely the reverse is true and it is the time in the month when our emotional truth speaks most forcefully. But know that if you let this truth out unprocessed at this time, you may cause more damage than you wish. If you feel it's okay for you, write or paint or talk it out first, before lashing out and hurting the feelings of those you love. But do not sacrifice your own health on this account; always try to keep a balance between honoring your own feelings and taking care of those around you. Educate your nearest and dearest to take your premenstrual irritability seriously, rather than belittling you and making PMS jokes. Your PMS is an attempt to bring emotional clarity. Remember this.

Energy movement, cleansing, and clearing This will help move any blocked psychological and emotional material. Exercise is key in balancing out the premenstrual time. Just make sure you do exercise that is fun for you. It is counterproductive, in the long run, to force your body to do things that your mind is not enjoying.

Supplements Vitamin B6 can be especially helpful in balancing premenstrual hormones. Vitamin B6 is a diuretic, and deficiency of this vitamin is often involved in pre-menstrual weight gain, bloating and associated sense of lethargy. Tension, anxiety and premenstrual acne also indicate the need for B6.

Diet Pay attention to your diet. Less salt, sugar and caffeine, more high-quality carbohydrates, like brown rice, whole wheat, root vegetables, pasta and honey.

Dysmenorrhea

Symptoms: pain and cramping before and during menstruation, sometimes accompanied by nausea.

Relaxation The number one remedy par excellence for cramps is to Lie Down. Relax. Let yourself enter the dreamy state of consciousness that is the gift of menstruation. Let go of "normal" life and domestic chores and work pressures. Put your feet up and chill out. Have I made myself clear?

Heat A hot water bottle or heat pad will also help. If you have severe cramps and heat makes them worse, go and have a check-up from your doctor.

Essential Oils Have a warm aromatherapy bath. Suitable oils include chamomile, clary sage, cypress, jasmine, juniper, marjoram, melissa, peppermint, rosemary. Follow your nose. Chamomile and melissa will calm you down, clary sage will cheer you up, and peppermint and rosemary will wake you up.

Herbs Cramp bark and the herbal mixtures made up by some of the women's herbal pharmacies.

Supplements Magnesium is a muscle relaxant and can help with cramps.

Cloth Pads Some women get worse cramps if they use tampons. Try letting your blood flow out unimpeded onto a nice flannel pad.

Inner Work Ask yourself what your womb is trying to tell you. How do you feel about having children? About your own creativity? About your love life? Be honest with yourself. This is the time to get to know your deepest dreams and fears, and to eliminate stuck emotions along with your menstrual blood. If tears come, let them out.

Medical Check-Ups Severe cramps should always be checked out by your doctor. They may indicate a chronic pelvic infection, or endometriosis.

Amenorrhea

Symptoms: not having periods, missing periods, having very light periods.

Treatment The first thing to say about this condition is that it is not good for you, and may make you more prone to osteoporosis in later life. Menstruating every month makes all kinds of hormonal mechanisms happen in your body that ensure your continued good health. If you miss more than two periods and you have been menstruating for more than two years, go and see your doctor and get a full checkup to try and understand why you have stopped menstruating. It is not unusual to miss periods in the first two years after you begin to menstruate, but thereafter is cause for concern.

Do whatever you can to get your periods going again, because the longer the body is paralyzed, as it were, in terms of the normal hormone function, the harder it is to get everything working properly again.

Diet and Exercise Amenorrhea is most commonly found in teenage girls and young women who exercise and diet to excess. It is a warning sign of anorexia. Ask yourself, very candidly: Are you exercising too much? Are you eating too little? These are the primary causes of amenorrhea. If you have been on an intensive diet and exercise program you may have lost perspective about what is normal and healthy, so ask your mother, a healthy friend or your doctor for advice. Remember, you can get addicted to exercise, and to not eating. Both create altered states of consciousness, and it may be the altered state that you are craving as much as the desire for extraordinary fitness or thinness. If so, find ways to experience altered states without damaging your body, such as meditation.

Inner Work If you are sure that neither excessive exercise or dieting is the cause, and your periods have just stopped for no apparent reason, look for the psychological factor. What happened in the month before your period stopped? It may have been something that doesn't seem significant enough to stop you menstruating, but it may have triggered an older pattern, perhaps around fear of being a woman, of growing up, of getting pregnant. For some reason your body has taken you out of the normal experience of being an adult woman. How do you feel about yourself as a woman? About menstruating? About your love life? About the possibility of becoming pregnant?

Light therapy When you stop menstruating it means you have stopped ovulating. You can stimulate ovulation by manipulating your exposure to light at night. At the full moon either keep your drapes or blinds open so that the light of the moon enters your bedroom, or leave a light on for the three nights the moon is at its fullest. The rest of the month, make sure there is no light at all in your bedroom.

Supplements Sometimes amenorrhea occurs because of a dietary deficiency such as zinc or iron. If you have been eating properly it is highly unlikely that you would have either of these, but if you are a young woman, especially in your teens, and you have been dieting, it's quite easy to get a deficiency because your body is still growing and needs a lot of nutrients on a regular basis.

Essential Oils: The following essential oils will help to stimulate menstruation: chamomile, clary sage, fennel, hyssop, juniper, lavender, marjoram, melissa, myrrh, pennyroyal, rose. Pick the scent you like the best and have an aromatherapy bath or massage at least once a day.

Irregular menstruation

Symptoms: when your cycle goes awry and the interval between periods becomes irregular, either shorter or longer than usual.

Food Avocado has a strong effect on the pineal gland and can help bring your cycle back to regularity. Eat at least half an avocado a day for a month.

Soya products have an estrogenic effect on the body, and that can stimulate more frequent ovulation. If you have a short cycle, try cutting out foods containing soya beans. Eating a lot of chicken heats the blood (in Chinese medical terms) and can shorten your cycle.

Light therapy Sleep with the light on at the time of the full moon, as described for amenorrhea, above.

Essential oils Clary sage, melissa, and rose will all help to stabilize your cycle.

Lifestyle Stress and accompanying tension can throw the cycle off. Try getting a regular massage to help you relax. Look at the way you are structuring your life and ask yourself: Is this too much pressure? How can I live in a way that is more fun? Am I trying to achieve in the outer world at the expense of my soul development?

Herbs If you think stress is a factor, try taking relaxing herbs such as chamomile, valerian or hops.

If you suffer from any of the above symptoms, especially if they are prolonged or severe, make sure you have a proper medical check-up with your primary healthcare provider.

If appropriate, look for a sympathetic holistic doctor in your area who can help you with natural medicine such as acupuncture, herbs or bodywork. Most menstrual complaints readily clear up, given the correct help.

PART FOUR

WAKING UP
TO THE POWER

THE STORIES
OF THREE WOMEN

In the winter of 1990-1991 I interviewed three women
who had had strong experiences with menstruation.
In the following chapters they tell their stories.

CHAPTER TEN

The Scientist: Wendy Alter

Wendy Alter was only thirty-four when she found a lump in her breast. It was cancer. Since graduating from college she had been a high-flyer with NASA, literally. Her ambition was to become an astronaut. As a chemist she had been exposed to toxic chemicals frequently during her adult life. But exposure to toxicity was only one of the causes that Wendy suspected had laid her open to cancer; another, equally insidious one, was her relationship to her femaleness.

"I started in a research position at NASA and gradually got more responsibility until I was managing large projects. I was in a very masculine-dominated world and had been ever since I could remember. In engineering classes there were very few women. I got an undergraduate degree in chemistry, and then I went back to school and I studied electrical engineering and computer science. Then I went to work for NASA, and when I'd been there for a few years I started doing graduate work in materials engineering. I was always around men. In my younger years I wished that I were a man. I hated being female; I hated it; I hated it.

My mother was a very, very confident woman who didn't want to be at home, didn't want to have anything to do with housework and children. She was professionally successful but she was of a generation where that wasn't quite respected and… well, she was respected, but people weren't quite sure if it was all right. She was a supervisor nurse, very successful in her work.

When I was a child I spent a lot more time with my father than I did with my mother. He spent a lot of time explaining things to me; he was very mechanically inclined and so that was a fun thing for me, and I think that's why I eventually ended up in engineering. I had a younger sister, and I have an older brother who is autistic.

When I reached my teens and I started to become noticeably female, my father stopped having anything to do with me, and this was painful for me. He started giving me some strange messages that boys don't like girls who are too successful and win races and things like that; it was a really painful, traumatic time. I was having my periods and I had terrible dysmenorrhea. My mother and sister had it too. I had very heavy flow, practically a hemorrhage, to the point where I would throw up – too much of a flow to wear a pad. It was terrible. And it was embarrassing because the school system completely denied that sort of thing: you were allowed to go and lie down at the nurse's station for one class period only, and other than that they just had no tolerance. I remember one time my sister had to be carried out by two guys, just as white as a sheet, and yet no one could talk about it.

It still annoys me that this is not a subject that can be discussed in mixed company, and often not among women either. When your friend gets a cold you usually get the whole story of how it developed and every minute of it, but when you're having your period, even if you're having terrible cramps, you have to pretend that everything's normal because you can't let anyone know. It's shameful to have your period. We all have a million stories about embarrassing incidents or mortifying experiences. And of course the doctors at that time all took the position that the pain was a psychosomatic problem caused by the fact that a female didn't feel good about being a female – that was the explanation that was given to me and it was hard to refute because indeed I didn't feel good about being a woman. When I got old enough to talk back, I started asking these doctors if it had ever occurred to them that maybe they had the cause and effect the wrong way round: if you had to go through that much pain every single month because of your gender wouldn't you come to resent your gender? It seems to me that their explanation was really weak.

I was so resentful when I was young, really resentful, because I was unusually intelligent and that was problematic, as a female. Advisors were always telling me that I should become a librarian, or a teacher. I really resented that. I did have a lot of dates and boyfriends, but I was resentful that things seemed to be easy for them. But at that time, I was an early feminist. I'm 38 now. My understanding of feminism was kind of wacky because what I wanted was the right to be treated like a man.

I had to come to the realization that there is something inherently valuable in the female by going all the way into the masculine, and I did that successfully. I had to prove to myself that I could do it, and prove to everyone around me that I could do it. And I was very successful, but I became aware that there was something seriously wrong. The working schedule is not natural – the idea that you work for the same amount of hours all the time, and you're supposed to be equally productive all the time, and you schedule your vacation three months in advance. It was so cut off from the real world.

My periods were a real bane to me when I was working. They were very, very irregular for many years and it seemed that my body had a mind of its own. It seemed to be trying to sabotage me, because my period would come early or late so that they happened during some major event. For example, I got to participate in NASA's weightless program – weightlessness by freefall in an aircraft. This was something I really wanted to do because I wanted to be an astronaut and this was a big step in the right direction. I was very ambitious from a young age. But the physiological training you take through the air force is very physically demanding. I had to go through the altitude chamber, where they pump out the atmosphere so you get to feel what it's like to be at twenty-six thousand feet without air, and they also put you through an explosive decompression. And of course, my period came during the training session. I was worried about whether it would have an adverse effect on me, to be menstruating at twenty-six thousand feet. But I didn't ask anyone about it; I just went ahead with the exercise.

There was one older woman that I had sort of latched onto as a mentor – she was a very male-identified woman also. I mentioned to her that I had my period, and she laughed and said that the same thing had happened to her and indicated that she had had some fears about what might happen going in and being depressurized. She hadn't said anything to anyone either.

Then I had my period again the very first time I flew a zero gravity mission. And when I had my period I'd become a little bit faint and light-headed – you know, things change – so to be in a very physically demanding situation like that and to have my period was awful. And every time, it was guaranteed to coincide with a physically demanding event. But my attitude was that it was essential never to let on to anybody that there would be any thing wrong with me and to go on, to be able to give a peak performance.

The years went by and I just started to feel kind of dead. The more successful I became, the more out of touch I felt. I felt like I was living a two-dimensional life somehow, as if I was some kind of cartoon character. Nothing seemed real any more. But it was really difficult to tear myself away because I had a big salary and everyone thought I was great and I was winning awards. But I wasn't happy. I became more and more unhappy and I couldn't even talk to anyone about it; what did I have to be unhappy about? It was a difficult time.

I had very few female friends. I worked around men. I got married during that time and we had a role-reversal marriage. My husband didn't work, he stayed home and he did all the cooking and shopping and house cleaning. After a while I did make a good female friend, and one day in a conversation with her and another woman, they mentioned how much they enjoyed having their periods. I was flabbergasted. It was so far from anything I had imagined. It had never occurred to me that there could be anything enjoyable about menstruating. That got me thinking. These were two very unusual women, very thoughtful women who had done a lot of inner work. I really respected them, and what they said caught my attention.

It took getting cancer to finally get me out of that situation. When I went through the ordeal with cancer I never even cried. In fact, when I received the diagnosis, my husband and I immediately went to the library and did a lot of research and found out everything there was to know and made decision trees.

It was all very rational, and I had no feelings; I couldn't feel. I was so used to not acknowledging feelings or giving them any attention or honoring them. All I could feel was this strange heaviness. That was the only way I could contact my feelings. I knew that wasn't helping, and I felt that it had to do with how I got cancer. There were plenty of other reasons too: I have a family history of breast cancer, and I had been working with carcinogenic substances for years.

The breast cancer was one of a series of illnesses I had that were all in my female organs, starting small and getting worse, I had cervical dysplasia a few months before the cancer was diagnosed. I had had a couple of surgeries for endometriosis a few years before. I finally sat down and said, "My body's trying to get my attention." It was as if I was trying to amputate anything of myself that was female.

I went ahead and did all the standard medical things that were recommended, even though I was pretty uncomfortable with it. I didn't feel I was in a position to explore any other options at that point. I carried on working. I was in Alabama; there was no alternative medicine there. And I didn't know anything about alternative methods of treatment anyway. I had various people write to me and say drink wheatgrass juice or something like that but at that point I wasn't prepared to do something like that. So I had the traditional treatments, but I wasn't entirely happy about it. I still suffer the side effects of the treatments. The chemotherapy is poison; you inject yourself with poison bad enough to kill the cancer but not quite bad enough to kill you. But your body knows, and when that poison goes in you feel poisoned and you feel weak. I still don't feel like I have my full strength back, and that's not from the cancer, it's from the treatment. Psychologically I had such a negative response to that treatment, and I know that attitude has a lot to do with one's health. Anyway I did what I felt I had to do at the time, and then I left my job.

My husband and I moved back to Washington, his home state. I pretty much spent the first year in shock. I didn't know what I was looking for; all I knew was that I wanted to get back in touch with my feelings. I started taking music lessons and art lessons. It was very difficult for me to do this. I started taking yoga; that was a revelation. I had no idea; I had completely underestimated what yoga was all about. I started to learn things about my body that I had never known.

My days now are very free of responsibilities. When we moved to Washington, my husband's desk-top publishing business was becoming successful, and so we did a turn-about since he hadn't worked in Alabama. He works at home, which has been a thorn in my side because I like to have a lot of completely quiet alone time, especially when I have my period. I never get that because he's always there; even when he's in another room in the house it's not the same – I still feel compelled to think about him and what he's doing and whether it's time for lunch yet. He's really worked hard to let me do what I've needed to do, and this has been a struggle for him too, but we both recognize that it is really obvious that around the time of my period strange things happen, and he is just as happy to avoid me at that time. So it hasn't been hard at all to work into a routine whereby I keep him posted and he gives me a wide berth, respectfully; he's always very compassionate. It's difficult to spend as much time alone as I want though because he feels threatened and neglected by this: I need a lot more time alone than he does so it's hard for him to understand sometimes. I need to find a retreat. I really want to be alone, but I want to stay at home, I don't want to go away. At home I have the things around me that I need for my creativity: my books, my computer. I don't feel domestic, I don't think about cooking much when I have my period; I'm not very hungry then.

I still have a lot of trouble with cramps and I have a medication that I take for it, but I've got to the point where I don't want to take it any more than I have to. I feel that I want to go ahead and have my period, even though there is pain associated with it. I don't want to just put chemicals into my body to deal with it. After the cancer treatments, I developed a real distaste for putting a lot of chemicals into my body, and I don't like the state that the pain medication puts me into.

I use that time as an excuse to do what I really want to do, which is usually just to go to bed. I love to read, so I take a stack of books, ideas that I'm working on at a given time, things that I want to mull over and sort of germinate. Our bedroom is in a tower room that has windows all around and we have a water bed, so it's really cozy. I just go up there and spend two days in bed and write and read.

At first I did it as an excuse; any excuse to read rather than to do chores around the house, which I hate, but it didn't take long at all for me to realize that as soon as I made a little room at that time amazing things were happening. I would just write prolifically and ideas would flood into my head, strong insights into things, and it would be a very positive experience. I realized that the negativity that I expressed sometimes was not inherent in having my period; it had to do with having to interact with people at that time. It was more annoyance at being taken away from what I really wanted to be doing rather than something inherent in the experience.

I decided about a year ago that I wanted to do a strict detoxification and I went to a nutritionist who put me on a very strict diet. After a month or so I had my period and I was out of my pain medication. I thought oh no, I'll just have to dig in and wait this one out, but I never did get cramps that month. It was the first time I really was able to recognize that there is some kind of dietary factor. But that diet was so restricted that I was getting weak and losing a lot of weight. I was unhappy with it, so I decided to discontinue it.

My poor body has really borne the brunt of whatever I wanted to do. When I had the chemotherapy they warned me that there was a 50% chance of being thrown into a premature menopause and at the time I was disappointed that this didn't happen – I would have been relieved. When I had endometriosis, I took a very powerful male hormone for a year during which time I had no periods; it was wonderful in terms of my career. But I realize now that even though I still have estrogen in my body, which increases the risk of breast cancer, I am really glad I haven't stopped menstruating because I never would have come to learn what a positive experience it can be.

Yesterday, I was thinking about this and I thought, yes, I have estrogen just coursing through my body and medically speaking it's dangerous to me. I decided to reject that whole idea. How can it be dangerous to me? I thought about all the wonderful things that estrogen does for me and how good it feels, and at that moment I could feel it in my body. I ended up doing this spontaneous meditation of gratitude towards my estrogen. It was a very good feeling. And I think if I took the time to do this on a regular basis a lot of my problems would go away. And the illnesses I have had might never have happened if I had respected my body.

Although NASA is a good equal opportunity employer, it is still run from a male perspective. There is a male way of making decisions and it wasn't until I had been there for ten years that I finally realized that I am different from these people. I can do that little logical thing that they do, but it doesn't feel right. There are some important things that they are leaving out.

There is another way of looking at and solving problems that's maybe more a female way. Taking in a lot of information and then leaving it alone – don't work on it, don't analyze it, don't try and draw a logical conclusion but let it all ferment – and the answer will come on its own. That's what women have to offer, and I find, from my personal experience, that it's a far superior way of coming to conclusions.

If you use the analytical model you can come to any conclusion you want, depending on what assumptions you choose to use, and that's one reason why so many bad decisions are made.

I have been really working on concepts of darkness and light; I had a dream and I woke up with this tremendous conviction that the light was suffocating the darkness, choking it off, and everything was terribly skewed and wrong because of that. This was a strange conclusion to come to, because in all the spiritual work I've been trying to do, light is always the good part. But I've come to realize that the darkness is equally good, and I wrote some things about the idea of the darkness; I'm thinking that that is where that fermentation happens. There's a certain violence and strangeness that comes from this extreme worship of the light without any darkness to balance it.

This year more than ever before I've been struck by ideas that are incredibly exciting to me, and have then come across other people having the same idea. Of course, this happens all the time in science; it's well documented: the same idea arises in different places simultaneously. Sometimes it comes in with such a force that it totally overwhelms me, some kind of outside force that takes over.

I have wanted to set up my life so that there are very few constraints on my time, so that when the inspiration comes I can be fully available for it. Now I'm becoming interested in coming back into the world again. It will be a creative work in itself to find a way of working that isn't excessively scheduled; we are so obsessed with that in this culture. A few months ago I had to do something during my period that I was committed to, and I was so miserable all the way through it, I was just so mad that I was there. My periods are regular now, so I plan in advance as much as I can. I have a chart and keep track so I can pretty well predict when it will come. And I suppose if it can schedule itself to come at inconvenient times, then there's no reason it shouldn't come at convenient times too."

CHAPTER ELEVEN

The Educator : Tamara Slayton

I interviewed Tamara at her home in Sebastopol, California, which then served as the headquarters for the Menstrual Health Foundation, a non-profit organization dedicated to providing education and resources about the positive and powerful aspects of menstruation. Her living room showed the evidence of her work, with baskets overflowing with cloth menstrual pads in different sizes and colors ranging from white to pink floral to bright red; bulletin boards covered with organizational data for classes and workshops; books on menstruation and related subjects.

As we talked it became clear that Tamara was a woman with a mission, who thought deeply about menstruation all her adult life. She first became aware of the deeper meaning of menstruation in 1974 when she was working with Jeannine Parvati Baker on the book Hygiea: A Woman's Herbal. Tamara went on to establish the MHF in 1983, as it became increasingly clear to her that work in this area was vitally important.

Tamara's pioneering and inspirational life was relatively short. She died in 2003 at the age of 53. For more information about her life and work, see the website, tamaraslayton.com.

"My mother is a hairdresser and has spent all her life around women, listening to women, counseling them, supporting them, being with them. So that was what I grew up with, that was my model of how women are in the world, and my mother really demonstrated the care of women. She didn't take care of herself in the process, and that's the part I have to undo, but she really was a model of a woman who listened to and cared deeply for other women.

I had a total lack of initiation into menstruation. I remember standing in the closet with my mother, and I had to be the adult because she was so embarrassed. I was scared but she was more so. After that came sexual activity that was totally unconscious, with no information, no support, and no one to talk to, resulting in pregnancy at the age of fifteen. I think that propelled me into working with women of all ages and helping them to become conscious. I was driven to do it because of the pain that was unintegrated. I've been working on integrating that pain, trying to find my son who was adopted, and really getting conscious of what happened and of what I lost. My grandmother got pregnant when she was seventeen and they whisked her out of the East to California. When I was fifteen and I got pregnant, my mother whisked me out of the town we were living in to another one, and so it was a secret thing.

When I was twenty-three I met Jeannine and began to become more conscious. It was towards the end of the back-to-the-earth hippie movement. I did a lot of primal therapy, tearing down ways of looking at things, and using psychedelics. There was a lot of breaking down to do. And I'm a survivor of sexual abuse, which is something that I'm working through now. This shows up in my classes all the time; at least seven of the current class have been abused. It comes up as soon as we begin to look at issues around caring for ourselves. It's very powerful work and it's very beautiful to watch someone reclaim her inner child, and see how that shows up premenstrually, how that vulnerability comes up very strongly. It's very powerful to start working with it from that point, and using it as part of the overall recovery.

I first began to think of menstruation as something powerful from spending time with Jeannine and teaching classes on fertility awareness with her and really starting to develop a whole new concept of what it meant to cycle. For Jeannine it was a little bit like second nature, it wasn't that she studied – she just came in with some information about menstruation. I lived with her for three or four years in community, and we talked about menstruation regularly and shared our dreams and discussed what happened for us each cycle.

I started changing my thoughts and the ways I spoke about myself, particularly premenstrually, and then I started just observing. I went into a witness mode, rather than judging or evaluating. I was very much into meditating so I had developed the skill of watching. I also started teaching a class of fertility awareness at the local junior college, and in that class it became real clear to me that most women did not like the fact that they bled, did not have a positive experience when they first started their menstruation, and were actually relieved when they got pregnant. So I was trying to teach them about fertility awareness and how to choose pregnancy consciously – and in some ways they were opting for an unconscious pregnancy because it relieved them of many things including menstruation. I began to see that there was something missing, and that if I was going to successfully teach fertility awareness I needed to include something around menstrual awareness.

The more I looked at it, the more I saw that the negativity is cultural. The entire culture is shame-based and dysfunctional around it. Around that time toxic shock syndrome happened, and, realizing how dangerous tampons could be, I became inspired to make natural pads.

A friend and I started working on what really needed to happen if women were going to become conscious of what they were wearing to absorb their blood and the deeper issues associated with that. So we created a non-profit educational corporation with profit-oriented activities in pad production. That was how the Menstrual Health Foundation started.

Part of this consciousness came for me out of struggling with what kind of birth control to use. I had changed my diet and lifestyle, but I was still using an IUD. I thought this is crazy – I had almost died from the IUD. I thought, well, there must be a way to relate to my fertility that doesn't risk my life, so I began to track my cycle, and I began to see how it is punctuated by these different hormone shifts.

It's my experience and the experience of the women I work with that the shift in consciousness arises when the shift in hormones occurs in the pre-menstrual time. In a healthy woman this will hit three or four days before she begins to bleed, and it typically results in a desire to withdraw into solitude or to communicate about ways she wants to restructure her life or relationships.

I don't see that as much during the bleeding time. When I hit my bleeding time I've usually settled into it, and there's a release of the tension that's been building up around that aspect of the creative dynamic. Before the bleeding I am really looking at things in fragments and pulling it apart, and then when it starts I begin to pull it all together.

It got emphasized for me because I came into this work with PMS. For women who are highly symptomatic, from day 14 they are already beginning to experience the premenstrual time and starting what we call the Kali period, starting to experience things falling apart and going out of control, in part because they are nutritionally deficient and suffer from a lack of exercise and excess stress. In healthy women it probably hits three to four days before they bleed.

It's a critically significant aspect of the female matrix and it takes one down into the darkness. Once you begin to bleed you begin to come back out. During the premenstruum the dream life is different. Childhood issues, struggling with things that happened when we were very young, rage in dreams, archetypes of Kali, the Black Madonna, dark goddesses, snakes, images of the dark – all that dark material that women have access to appears in dreams, and if we can claim that dark side, we can work with it. It tends to show up in dress too: women prefer to wear darker colors in the premenstruum.

To me it's a process of sorting through what am I being told is real about this time and what *is* real to me. When you are able to express rage in a safe and nurturing environment then it does begin to slough off, and you get down to the next level of communication. There's a very ancient body of information available there. The first thing I work with is women to be okay with this rage. There is a distinction between the crisis stage when one fears losing control – focusing on what is wrong with being female, attacked by one's own body, isolated and despairing –

and then moving into the observation stage of noticing that those are the cultural distinctions of a much deeper phenomenon.

The nutritional aspect of PMS is also very important. It's very hard to gather wisdom if your B vitamins are depleted and if you are strung out on sugar and caffeine. Then you are dealing with the breakdown every month rather than the integration of the wisdom. We eat too much fragmented food that has been over-processed. But it's very hard to get whole foods in a convenient way. Women are on the run, on the go; it's hard to get your hands on something that is quick, nutritious and affordable.

Our soil is very depleted, which is really another metaphor of what's happened to the feminine. So we're faced with poor quality food and the fact that we can't get it, and then when we do get it we eat it so fast we can't assimilate it. With the amount of stress we experience in our lives we need good nutrition. I think that we do need vitamin supplements and most women can't afford them. If you are going to gather the wisdom of the cycle then you have to have a good diet.

This wisdom is available not only during the premenstruum and the period but also at fertility. There's a whole wisdom that's being generated with each cycle – the creation and the destruction aspect each balancing the other – and to be able to listen to that inward conversation that's going on about how I'm living, how I'm conducting my life, I have to be healthy enough to be able to get to it, otherwise I'm just repairing all the time. And that may be where the woman needs to be, but if you can get her to lie down and really take care of herself, that she may be able to get to that deeper understanding of her life which her cycle will give her if she'll just start listening. Ignoring that inner conversation stems from the dishonoring of the feminine in the culture – not just of women but of the whole need to go inward and gestate and be in darkness. So the one who carries that the most, which is the female, suffers.

There is a rhythm to it and if you watch it you notice the rhythm, and then you begin to trust it. Through witnessing every cycle and seeing that there is a rhythm to your psychology, your spirituality, your physicality, you begin to see: Ah yes, I do go inward, things do get dark, I really need to feel safe in order to let things fall apart, and then I know I'll come out of it and I'll be on top of the mountain and full of fertility and life will be bright and shiny again and I'll want to socialize and I'll want to be close to people, and then I'll want to go back down again. The more I observe that, the more I trust it, and the more I gather the fruits of both aspects of the cycle.

During my premenstruum and my period I tend to do a lot more journal writing and a lot more assessing of what am I doing in my life now: Is this really what I want to be doing? What do I want to complete? What is it that I am avoiding completing? I usually make a list of who I need to say something to, what I need to communicate, and what I am afraid to say to them, and then I go about doing those things.

So I'm doing a lot of processing, a lot of grieving, a lot of letting-go work. All this tends to be premenstrual. After I bleed I'm usually in my room, doing some kind of artistic process, meditating, praying, writing. I try to get in here at least one night and sleep in here on my own, which is challenging with the kids and my boyfriend, but more and more it's where I find myself. I tend to do more artwork, more work around the transformational Goddess: Kali dolls, witch dolls, things like that. I soak my pads in a bowl or a teapot, and the whole pad thing is a ceremony in itself: taking care of your blood, finding your pads, putting them back afterwards. For me that's very important: I had no rhythm as a child. I try to water my plants with my blood. And sometimes I don't do any of that stuff; sometimes it's all I can do to bleed and keep my life going. It's such a conflict now for women, with all the responsibilities that we have as single mothers, to really incorporate that kind of life. It's very challenging. We don't want to create a whole new set of things we have to do. So I avoid beating myself up because I don't withdraw every month.

It is also a good time to think about how I earn a living. If a woman starts listening premenstrually, she usually runs into her heart's desire and then she has to figure out how to get it. This is a good part of the goodies that are available in menstrual and premenstrual consciousness.

I assert that what we are working with here is a matrix. With menarche you meet your wisdom, and then with your monthly bleeding you practice your wisdom, and then at menopause you become the wisdom."

CHAPTER TWELVE

The Priestess : Hallie Iglehart Austen

Hallie Iglehart Austen is a priestess. One of the early leaders of the women's spirituality movement, she has dedicated her life to the return of the sacred feminine into modern life. She teaches the techniques of earth-centered ritual to groups of women, and leads celebrations at equinoxes and solstices and other holy days for women, men, and children. Her first book, Womanspirit, *came out in 1983, and influenced a generation of feminists hungry for a sense of woman-as-divine, and whose spiritual yearnings could find only male gods and leaders in the established religions. Her second book,* The Heart of the Goddess – Art, Myth and Meditations of the World's Sacred Feminine, *was published in 1991.*

When I interviewed her, Hallie was living in the hills above Point Reyes in Northern California, in a round house that sits in a hollow in the land, surrounded by tall fir trees. She migrated here from Berkeley in 1986 to write and teach and live close with the earth. Her writing room was a small, cozy room at the top of a spiral staircase, with windows on three sides looking out at the swaying treetops and the blue blur of the ocean in the distance. It seemed fitting that she live and work in this beautiful, still wild part of the planet, surrounded by earth and water, trees and sky.

After graduating from Brown University in the late sixties, she traveled to Asia and was very attracted to the Tibetan Buddhists she met in Dharamsala in the northern Indian Himalaya. She studied with them, wintering in the high mountains and learning their ritual and meditation practices. In between visits to India she would return to the States where she became involved with the growing feminist movement.

"It was a split time for me," she recalls. "On the one hand I

*was very involved with the feminist movement, and then I would
spend time in India studying what was in many ways a male-
dominated spiritual tradition."*

*Eventually the split became overwhelming, and she moved
back to the United States to see if she could discover a sense of the
spiritual that enhanced rather than contradicted feminism.*

"I decided to move to San Francisco, where so many exciting
things were happening, and I continued my work with the
Feminist Health Center. There the relationship between the
patriarchy and women's health became very clear to me. I didn't
have my period for a year and a half after taking birth control
pills. Now it is something that I really guard and treasure because
of having lived without it, and I felt that it was really something
that the patriarchy robbed me of.

It was quite a revelation to start working at the Feminist Health
Center and see what these pills had done to my body. When I was
taking them in the mid to late sixties it was just considered
wonderful if you could get them; huge doses of hormones and no
one was questioning it at all.

The first time I bled after that year and a half was very
dramatic. I was cross-country skiing up in Yosemite. I was off by
myself and I squatted to pee in the snow and this red fell on the
snow. It was the first time I'd seen my menstrual blood in a year
and a half. It was very beautiful. I remember that moment, even
though it was seventeen years ago – it was so visual. I was very
happy because I'd been doing several things to try to get my
period back. At the same time I had cervical dysplasia so it was
even more of a sign that my health was better, because I got rid
of the dysplasia and got my period back. Because of that
experience I've really treasured my period.

I remember in 1969 being furious with a lover, a man. We'd
been lovers for quite a while, and he wouldn't make love with me
when I had my period. I felt good about my menstrual blood but
I don't remember thinking of it as sacred until I started getting into
women's spirituality and the Goddess."

In 1975, Hallie and several co-priestesses created a menstruation ritual in Oregon for 200 women.

*   *   *

"We did the blood ritual in a big meadow under a full moon. The main point was painting ourselves with menstrual blood and saying really affirmative things about menstruation. When we created the ritual, the idea was to counteract the negative ideas about menstruation. Doing that ritual was wonderful and celebratory. I'm sure in retrospect now that it really grounded me in my body in a way that I wouldn't have been otherwise; that's always an ongoing process of course. (See Appendix i for recommendations regarding HIV and the use of menstrual blood in ceremony.)

I've been through various stages in my relationship with my bleeding. I tried using sponges but they didn't hold enough for me. I can't remember when the shift of not using tampons came; probably when toxic shock syndrome came out.

I don't always know enough to be able to plan around my bleeding; sometimes I have a workshop scheduled months in advance. I feel like I've gone through many phases with my bleeding, Certainly there was a phase of really loving it and honoring it and opening up with wonder to something that has been denied for so long. After it became regular, I had severe cramps and so that was a whole other teaching and journey: learning to deal with that pain that demanded that I pay attention to it. I honor my period as best I can.

I try to bleed on the ground at some point. It was a way for me to connect with the earth even when I lived in Berkeley; if I could go out and bleed onto a little plot of earth it was a way to ground even when I was living in concrete. That felt like a very important link and it's something I recommend to women who live in cities, if they can, just to take a moment to bleed onto the ground. Your cells are blending with the earth; you are connected to the earth by your blood being there. Here I'm surrounded by the earth so it's not so much of an issue. For me bleeding on the earth is an opportunity to experience it in a natural way. Sanitary pads aren't too natural but they are convenient, whereas bleeding on the earth, that's real. It's important for me to tap back into how people lived in another time. That may sound romanticized but when you live outdoors you don't have to worry about bleeding on things.Native Americans bled on moss.

What's changed for me more recently is allowing myself to do whatever I want to do on the first day of my period, whether it's going off a big hike, hanging around, or working. I'm allowing myself to be spontaneous, and if I don't do that I get cramps. I know why so many women in offices get menstrual cramps: it's because they are sitting at desks. If you can lie down or walk or whatever, it really helps a lot.

I think of the first day as the strongest time, I think of it as a transitional time, the time between bleeding and not bleeding. I feel something beginning the day before, a lot of things are going on in my body at a cellular level. Sometimes it's also the second day that is very powerful. I feel most respectful whenever the flow is heaviest. When you're sitting there bleeding, bleeding, bleeding, it's hard to keep a normal schedule because this thing is happening which is quite miraculous and also requires attention.

A friend of mine told me of a woman she knew who, when she was menstruating, could always tell when blood was about to come. I was very struck by that. It made me want to be more aware and now, when I start to feel the blood come, I go outside. It's partly environmental – I use fewer pads – but it's also paying attention to the fact that blood is coming out of my body. I stop what I am doing and let it happen. I see menstruation as a Zen practice, as a monthly practice. Again, because I didn't have my period for so long, I learned to watch it more because it was important; watching it, asking myself what is it doing, like the birds or the sky, watching it do its dance. This watching may have come out of a need to do with my health, but now it's almost like this being that enters my body, and I watch it do its dance for those five days. Attention can be a key thing for women reclaiming their cycles.

The last few years I have noticed extreme sexual energy

around ovulation and menstruation. I feel myself particularly a priestess when I'm bleeding: it reminds me of my connection with all my sisters, all our mothers. It is something so basic and yet so big, so dramatic. It's amazing. Small wonder that whole ceremonies are based around it. For the Apache and several other Native American tribes the most important ceremony is the girls' puberty rites. In India, there is a spring that flows with iron oxide after the monsoon rains. People from all over make pilgrimages to this spring in Kamakhya, Assam, and drink the red water as the menstrual blood of the Earth Mother, the Goddess.

One of the most profound things for us Euro-Westerners to comprehend is that for some traditional peoples, menses is a time of power. If we could just get that, a lot of things would change: the work schedule, our attitudes toward women, sicknesses, more conscious birthing. Everything would change.

The alchemical process that takes place within us means that for women, our spirituality is internalized, and that perhaps it comes more naturally that we understand transformative processes. We know that it's true, we know that it's possible, we know that we can create this miracle in our bodies: birth, lactation, menstruation. That connects women up with the life force, more in the sense that we know it in our bodies that this happens, so it enables us to be more life-affirming because we create life. I think we have more acceptance through our bodily processes that things happen without our controlling them. We are more accepting of mystery. Menstruation just happens, it happens through us, we don't do anything to make it happen.

What we've lost in this culture is a sense of awe. I think that when we reclaim our sense of awe about menstruation, about blood, about the cycles of the moon, of our fertility, of the incredible changes that go on in our bodies, then we will be able to reclaim our sense of awe about the universe, because to me the menstrual cycle is a microcosm of the universe. So instead of one's lover being turned off by menstruation, one's lover can bow to it from every cell, with deep feeling.

We can recreate that sense of awe in the natural world by doing rituals, either alone or together. I think that because we don't have puberty rituals, we stay adolescents in some way. There has to be a reason why cultures have puberty rites. I see rituals and cycles as opportunities for letting go, for renewal and purification. Rituals are all about letting go of the old and making space for the new because we live on a planet of cycles. That's why menstruation is so important as we reclaim the true cyclical nature of life on this planet."

PART FIVE

LIVING YOUR POWER

CHAPTER THIRTEEN

Menstruation, Relationships and the Family

Deciding to have a deeper relationship with your bleeding means not only changing your relationship with yourself, but also shifting the ways in which you relate with others. It's one thing to sidle off alone into some quiet time, and it's another step to say to someone else, "I need to be alone now to be with myself; I have my period".

You don't have to do it all at once. If you are concerned that you will meet opposition from your partner and family, try working first with yourself and identifying the parts in you that are against you experiencing your bleeding, that are against the idea of it being a powerful time. You may well find an inner voice that tells you that you are wasting your time, that it is merely a biological function, that being a woman is simply a messy business and that you should just get on with it and experience it as little as possible. Get to know your conditioning and your biases. If it feels right, try engaging the conflicting voices in a dialogue and see how they interact. Encourage these voices to come out with their worst, and then see if there is a natural tendency for them to begin relating a little easier. Compromise may begin to emerge. The conventional voice may say, "Well, it's okay for you to meditate more but just don't think about bringing those cloth pads into the house." In time, as you experience the sense of wholeness that comes from living your bleeding time more fully, these conflicts will iron out, and your conventional part will be increasingly prepared to change.

When you feel you know your inner conflicts a little more, it will be easier to risk being unusual with other people. It will also be much more likely that they will feel at ease with what you are doing. Our friends and loved ones are mostly very sensitive to our own inner conflicts. Many arguments and relationship difficulties are the result of unrecognized inner battles.

Underlying tensions in your relationship will tend to be exposed during the premenstruum and during menstruation. If you and your partner are open to working through difficulties and dedicated to working on an honest, open, equal relationship, you can both come to deeply value the natural tendency of the menstrual cycle to cut through politeness and convention and to reveal problems early, before they become major relationship messes.

WANTING TO BE ALONE

As Wendy Alter said in Chapter 10, what she wants most is to be left entirely alone when she is bleeding.

Susun Weed, a well-known herbalist, said, "Visionary states of consciousness are more accessible when I am menstruating, if I provide myself with that intention and the place where I can freely experience that. I need privacy and quiet and not to feel compelled to respond to anyone else's needs but my own. If I have the safe space of the moon-lodge, then I find that it's easier for me to shift my consciousness." [1]

I have had the same experience: that if I can spend some time alone in peace and quiet, insight comes.

WANTING TO BE CLOSE

Some women find that rather than desiring time alone when they bleed, they have a greater need for reassurance and closeness. They feel vulnerable and in need of cuddles. Women may be more susceptible to feeling rejected at this time, particularly in the light of a culture which has rejected the bodily processes of the female in so many ways.

RELATIONSHIPS WITH MEN

Many women live with a man: a father, husband, son or boyfriend. Or if you live alone, you may work with men during the day. It's unusual in this culture to be completely apart from men when we are bleeding. So how can the sexes coexist at a time when in many traditions, women have gone apart from men?

One way is by the genders picking up some of each others' process. This is what is happening in our contemporary world: the roles that define men and women have blurred significantly.

A man who is in touch with his female side is much easier to be with when you are bleeding than a man who is very masculine. I use these terms with caution. Another way of saying this would be that a man who values the rhythm of his body and is able to articulate and experience his feelings is going to be easier to be around when you yourself are in a deep menstrual feeling state. A man who lives more in the traditional mold of the male – stoic, cut off from feeling, linear, literal – will be much harder to be with if you decide to go further into your menstrual experience.

Many women find that when they delve deeper into the menstrual mysteries they become uninterested in household chores while they are bleeding, or shortly before. If this is the case with you, then it's going to be crucial how much your partner can pick up the cooking and cleaning and childcare.

He needs to be able to take care of himself, and also to accept that for a few days every month you are taking care of yourself and may not be so available. This demands more sensitivity than men have traditionally given women in our culture; to be less demanding in terms of food, empathy, sex and social activities.

This trend of men picking up a wider range of feeling, and women going out more into the world, may be part of an overall shift in human consciousness away from a rigid experience of the self through gender. However, we have to be careful that technology and the rapid pace of modern life don't take us away from our centers, away from the knowledge of our bodies. In a male-dominated world, women's reality and experience suffers, and the loss of tribal identity and pride in gender manifests itself in the home as much as anywhere.

How well you, your partner and your bleeding get along together depends a good deal on the level of intimacy in the relationship. If you are able to talk deeply together about your feelings than you stand a good chance of being able to incorporate conscious menstruation into your domestic life. Some men enjoy the deepening of relationship and awareness that comes from the woman being able to really go into herself during her period. One couple I talked to told me that they have experienced highly spiritual times together during her period in which insight has come to both of them.

If the man in your life is an unconscious misogynist this may well show up more at menstruation than at any other time, because this is a time when the woman is most obviously female (and during pregnancy, of course). Ignoring or despising menstruation is one of the ways that misogyny manifests itself. And it's not only women who create fights around menstruation; men do as well. They will do this especially if they have a bias against slower dreamy energy, altered states, intuition, the release and expression of feelings, and the other states that constellate around menstruation.

How women view themselves and are viewed affects men too. It might look, on the face of it, that men have had the upper hand for the past few thousand years, but that is only true from a certain perspective. Both men and women have gained and suffered from the imbalances of patriarchal society. Men have also been separated from their bodies and from their feelings, and from the pleasure and healing made possible by relationships based on co-operation rather than hierarchy and dominance.

Imagine a world in which men and women worked together to develop the sense of inner peace that comes from sitting still for a couple of days once a month. In which men supported women to spend a few days in peaceful quiet. A world in which menstrual blood was once again a magical fluid with a power to nurture new life. A world in which menstruation was understood to be the Sabbath of women: a natural space within one moon's cycle for retreat, introversion and inner work, from which women emerge like the new-born moon itself, renewed, the old skin shed.

RELATIONSHIPS WITH WOMEN

There are many instances in cultural lore of women menstruating together in synchrony, and many women that I have spoken with have reported strange experiences of cycles changing to fit with co-workers, friends and lovers. Current research indicates that it is through smell – through sensing pheromones – that women pick up on each other's cycles and adjust accordingly. This phenomenon has particularly been observed in female dorms and in women's offices, and some women notice it in their family too.

The first time I experienced menstrual synchrony was on a school trip to Bavaria. I was fifteen, and assigned to a small group of seven fifteen- and sixteen-year-olds. For two weeks we traveled in the same train compartment and slept in the same hotel room. We were rarely out of each other's sight. We all began our period on the same day, about ten days into the trip, and at a time that was off-cycle for four of us. Since then I have experienced countless examples of this automatic blending of cycles that happens to women who spend a lot of time together.

Women often remark on the seeming strangeness of menstruating together. We are taught to think of ourselves as individuals, and menstrual synchrony is a powerful reminder of our tribal and animal nature. Menstruating together can be a strong bonding experience for women, creating an intimacy of being in the same altered state at the same time. The knowledge that our bodies shift cycle so that we are in harmony creates a feeling of sisterhood that can run deeper than our conscious sense of relationship with one another. The idea of the menstrual hut, a place where women go to menstruate, is very attractive to many women. The thought of having some company and being "in it together" is appealing.

From talking with women who are in relationships with

women, I have learned that there are several aspects to menstruating together. All the lesbian couples I spoke with have experienced a significant level of synchrony; one couple I know begin menstruating within an hour of one another. This gives a great feeling of being understood by your partner, and can be powerfully bonding. On the downside it can also mean that, as the closely synchronous couple told me, "the week before is hell", as both women have PMS at the same time. It demands consciousness on the part of both women to be able to process the feelings that come up at this time, together, and in ways which take care of each other. This makes it a potentially powerful time for experiencing altered states together as well as for processing issues in the relationship.

SEX AND MENSTRUATION

I have witnessed many heated discussions on this topic, and have concluded, entirely unsatisfactorily, that there are two types of women: those for whom menstrual sexuality is anathema, and those who absolutely love it. Whether you like the idea of it or not clearly depends on your own disposition, and on your partner. However, that said, I do think that you are dealing with powerful energy when you have sex during menses, and that it's sensible to be careful around that energy.

In the Tantric tradition, sex during menstruation is seen as particularly special, involving the mixing of the red and the white, the blood and the sperm, and giving the possibility of alchemically transforming the sexual partners. In "The Spirit of Intimacy", Sobonfu Somé says that, "During menstruation, sacred sexuality can happen with a woman depending on the kind of energy that exists between partners. The man must work at raising his energy to match that of the woman. If not, he could suffer from such an encounter. He could become disempowered." [2]

Menstruation and the Family

A woman's reproductive years are often dominated by the needs of others. Having a time of solitude apart from the demands of the family is a necessary balance. It is a time when the giver can reinforce her sense of self and get to know herself away from the needs of the family or workplace.

Many women find that they become significantly less interested in domestic chores, particularly cooking, when they have their period. The old taboos that women should not touch food when they were bleeding may have had their roots in an earlier awareness that women simply don't want to cook then, and a recognition that this is not a time for domestic work, but a time for one's own work. Likewise the Jewish restriction against eating cooked food on the Sabbath has its origins in the Sabbath's ancient connection to the New Moon and to menstruation and to the custom of women not having to cook when menstruating.

For the Deese family of Springfield, Oregon, becoming aware of menstrual power has led them to change their family life:

> About two years ago we began to establish a moon-time practice of relieving my wife from most domestic chores, mostly from food preparation. This brought moon-time into the working realities of everyone in the family, by requiring some mutual responsibilities that our young ones enjoy. The "inconvenience" requires adjustments which are beautiful openings for teaching and discussion.[3]

For many women, especially mothers, time alone is hard to come by. Creating a family pattern whereby mother gets a break when she has her period allows a crucial rebalancing to occur. Menstruating is not always about resting; sometimes it's about working and activity too. It is a great time for working creatively on what you love best, going for a hike in the woods, writing letters, watching the sky. It's a time for yourself, whatever you want to do. Sometimes it is hard for women to get in touch with what they need and want for themselves, as so much of their attention is bound up with the needs of others, particularly if they have children. Your period is a great time to practice getting in touch with your own needs.

CHAPTER FOURTEEN

Bleeding with the World

Just as our ancestors honored woman's ability to create humans from her womb and feed them from her breast, they also honored the Earth as the Great Mother who nourishes us and from whose body we are all created. It is clear that in order to save ourselves – not to mention fulfill our true potential – we must honor Nature, the Goddess, and women.

Hallie Iglehart Austen [1]

Menstruation, the Feminine and the Earth are all linked. The ways in which we perceive and experience menstruation have a ripple effect on how the feminine in general is perceived and experienced. If we are to find a way to live on this planet that is ecologically viable, we must reintegrate the feminine aspects of life in ways that at the moment still seem weird and bizarre to most people. One of the fundamental ways this necessary shift can take place is through gaining greater consciousness of the vital importance of the menstrual cycle as a fundamental rhythm in all our lives.

Chris Knight, in *Blood Relations: Menstruation and the Origins of Culture*, argues that the menstrual cycle was a crucial element in the establishment of the earliest human cultures. His theory, now accepted by a large body of evolutionary theorists and anthropologists, states that the earliest social structures were organized around the menstrual cycle, and that this organization was instigated by women in order to protect children and provide sufficient food for pregnant and nursing mothers, thus ensuring the survival of the human race.

We are now at a significant junction in the history of humankind, and as Knight points out, it is time once again to embrace the potential of menstruation for creating culture. As for the urging of modern feminists for even further denial of the reality of menstruation, Knight makes the irony of the situation clear: "only an extremely *masculinist* and *non-periodic* culture could impose its one-sided constraints so deeply as to make women conclude that it was they – but not men – who would have to suppress and deny their own biology as the condition of feeling liberated ... cultural liberation *ought* to give women the chance (where they wish to) to validate and derive social pride, status and power from uniquely female experiences such as childbirth and menstruation". [2]

When women are able to live in harmony with their natural cycles, their health improves and the balance of their lives is restored. When women are at peace with their fundamental rhythms, relationships between men and women improve, and cultural life stabilizes. When men and women can live in approximate harmony, they naturally want to care for the people and things around them. The earth is honored and properly stewarded, and people feel grounded and secure.

MENSTRUATION AND THE WORLD

The personal work you do premenstrually and during your period has a benefit for everyone. As the great spiritual traditions teach, even one awake individual can create harmony and awareness in the world around them. Our inner work is also work for the world. Women menstruating with insight feed that knowledge into the collective of humankind. This insight can also come from nonfocused thinking. The natural tendency of menstruation to provoke a diffused state of awareness means that it is an excellent time for dreaming and receiving guidance – guidance that can inspire and inform the world around us.

The Dalai Lama, one of the world's most eminent and forthright proponents of world peace, has spoken about the relationship between world peace and inner work. The creation of world peace is dependent on each individual's ability to experience inner peace.[3] The peace that is available to women, especially at the end of the period, is a built-in opportunity to experience a deep peace that then translates out into the surrounding world.

Being a Strong Woman in the World

In many ways, women need to be tough these days. We have to drive our own cars, earn our own money, take out our own garbage, raise children alone. This toughness and independence has become part of our survival, but it is also something that we choose, because it brings us more autonomy in our private lives and more power in the world. Yet in order to survive, and to live our power more fully, we don't have to become tough in the way that men are tough. We can use our toughness to draw our own boundaries, state our own needs, and create lifestyles that respect our cyclical body patterns. We can create a world in which it is a pleasure to have a period, in which each is free to menstruate in her own way, a world in which the first blood of young women is greeted with joy and pride. The world needs our strength, but it needs the strength of Women, not the pseudo-strength of pseudo-men.

The world needs the wholeness of women; it needs women with healthy wombs who know their own needs and can express their feelings and their wisdom. One of the ways women keep healthy is by taking time out, and by honoring their natural rhythms. There is growing evidence that working women are hit hard by the stress of modern life. There is a link between overwork and premature menopause. Under long-term stress, the adrenals burn out, in turn affecting the whole endocrine system and the production of estrogen. When estrogen stops being produced, women go into menopause. This is why shock and sudden grief can create premature menopause overnight.

With women suffering from work-related stress, menopause doesn't happen overnight, but it is coming on earlier and earlier in our society. A woman working in a high-powered job, in a male reality which doesn't allow for the cyclical nature of female physiology, is under additional stress for the few days every month when she would rather be resting or puttering about. Instead she carries on just the same, tearing around Manhattan or London or Chicago, and as she rushes around while the blood drips down, her adrenal glands attempt gamely to cope with the stress put on her system by this lifestyle. Chronic fatigue syndrome is an illness also caused by adrenal burnout, and the classic patient is a woman in her thirties or forties with a demanding lifestyle. We have to ask ourselves whether it is worth burning ourselves out and going through premature menopause in order to fit in with a way of life that is often quite insane as far as the female body is concerned.

In general, I recommend taking time out from work if you can when you have your period, especially on the first day or two when the bleeding is heaviest. If you have to go to work then take your menstrual energy consciously into the workplace. Allow more spaciness, intuition and slowness in your attitude at work. Our workspaces have been too dominated by linear thinking, by a mentality of striving. Take pride in the state that your period takes you into and change the office; don't let the office change you and create inner anguish, PMS and cramps. Don't let people rush you; do inner work on your tendency to hurry yourself.

The Return of the Feminine and the Healing of the Planet

We live at a time of increasing awareness of the female, when feminine values are being returned to the world. The world needs the creativity and compassion of women like it may never have needed it before. It needs women's particular and peculiar abilities to draw down the energy of the universe and manifest it on the planet. Women, by virtue of their biology, have an automatic link to the Great Mother. If they choose to tune into her through their wombs, they can access knowledge for the good of all.

This increased capacity for self-reflection and insight is not only significant for the individual woman but also for her partner and family and the larger community around her. Society as a whole unconsciously benefits (and could benefit a lot more) from the wisdom garnered by women who experience their bleeding with awareness. By becoming aware of this power and potential, we could stabilize our social fabric to a far greater degree. We can only speculate how much disharmony in family life is caused by women not paying attention to their natural rhythms. Many tribal peoples, such as the Cherokee, recognize that the menstruating woman is performing a function of cleansing and centering not only for herself but also for her family, and therefore for the whole tribe.

The changing status of women in society offers great hope for the re-integration of female perspectives into mainstream thinking. The influence of women is already being felt politically in the ecology and peace movements. Menstruation is an integral part of the development of women's spirituality, both at the individual and collective levels. For women as individuals, the acceptance of the value and power of menstruation is a key to our ability to access the Goddess within. Collectively, all aspects of womanhood need now to be acknowledged for their highest potential. The denial of female wisdom has contributed to our present state of potential annihilation through nuclear warfare, and the threatened poisoning not only of our own species, but also of many other species living on the planet.

It is only a short leap to the conclusion that the denigration of menstruation and the denial of its power arose out of fear and envy by male priests and rulers who wanted all the power to themselves. Where the power struggle between the sexes originated is open to speculation, but I prefer to assume that our experience of patriarchy has had a long-term evolutionary purpose. It appears likely that before this patriarchal period there flowered a matriarchy, which died just as this present culture will die.

Rather than look back with longing to an imagined golden age of Goddess worship, we can look forward to a future where the whole of the Feminine and the whole of the Masculine are given the opportunity to flourish. This is a utopian dream, but it is a good place to aim our sights, as a culture. Sometimes we get caught in the nightmare of the collective, swept up in horrendous news reports of atrocities perpetrated all over the globe, made anxious by the knowledge of nuclear weapons testing, the destruction of the rain forests, and the heartless mutilation of our fellow creatures in the name of science. It pays to have a strong positive dream to counterbalance this horror, and to be ceaselessly pouring one's energy towards that dream of hope in the future, borne out of the knowledge of the essential magnificence of the dance of life and death.

The return of the feminine and the healing of the planet are intricately intertwined. We cannot have the change in the macrocosm that we know is essential for survival of life on the earth, without a parallel shift in the microcosm. For example, the recycling of household waste is a relatively minor achievement compared to getting major industries to stop polluting rivers or governments to stop nuclear testing, but it is nonetheless extremely important as a method of consciousness-raising and giving individuals ways to contribute to the safer ecology of the planet.

There is a strong relationship between our attitudes to our bodies and our attitude to the larger body – the planet Earth. It is not simply our behavior towards literal waste that needs to change, but also our attitude toward our bodies and their "waste". When menstruation is called a curse and suppressed as much as possible, then we are wasting a precious aspect of life. We are missing the point that the experiences inherent in the female have a value, a value which goes beyond the limits that twentyfirst-century Western society has allowed.

The political and social impact of our collective denial of the power of the menstrual cycle should not be underestimated. Acknowledging the levels of our disgust at our bodies and at the nature of femaleness is unpleasant, but this is vital to unraveling the threads that patriarchal culture has wound around our freedom as women, as human beings. Our throats have been strangled by these cords of self-disgust, as we stand by in horror and watch unnecessary wars fought, watch our sons killed and our daughters left without husbands, watch innocent people killed by bombing and by other horrendous means.

Behind this madness is the fact that women don't believe in themselves, and don't trust their own instincts enough to stand up and say, "*No*. My children will not die in this carnage. You will *not* destroy my family, my home, my town, my city, my country".

The essential nature of the female is not valued in this culture, and so we lack the confidence to stand up and exercise our power because we have largely forgotten what female power truly is. It has been debased into manipulation and acting behind the scenes, usually to aggrandize the husband. Or we see it in women acting more like men than men do.

One of the ways that genuine female power develops is through the careful gathering of self-knowledge and awareness through monthly meditation and retreat at the time of the bleeding. Female power is patience borne out of the experiences of gestation and child-rearing: nurturing an unseen embryo for nine months, sitting for hours nursing, rocking a restless baby in the middle of the night. Female power is female wisdom, and female wisdom resides in the body and is manifested by the experiences of the female body.

In a society which does not respect such qualities as awareness, sensitivity, patience and the ability to nurture, women don't respect these qualities either. They tend to skate with resentment over those times in their lives when those qualities would be ingrained into them, if they were available to receive them. If all women honored their bleeding and went into retreat every month, practicing rituals designed to increase self-awareness and self-love, the world would be a better place.

Men would discover their nurturing side as they took over the responsibility of childcare and the home for those few days a month; children would be relieved the burden of an irritable and tired mother who really would much rather be putting her feet up with a good book, and they would also benefit from relating with other adults. Above all, women's processes would once again be recognized as having an intrinsic value. Just as the body miraculously produces milk to feed the baby after it is born, so the body somehow produces wisdom in the psyche during menstruation, if it is given the space. Women don't have to *do* anything. In fact the less they do the better. It is more a case of sitting reasonably still for a while, and letting wisdom happen.

If women meditated every month, think how clear their minds would be when they emerged from their retreat. At that moment the leaders of the community should go to them and ask, "What should we do about this or that problem?" and listen to the clear-minded and heartful response that they would receive.

Imagine for a moment that there is a group of women who are nationally, perhaps internationally, recognized for their wisdom and for their ability to channel the wisdom of the collective. Perhaps some of them are crones who are past the age of menstruation, and some of them are still menstruating. When there is a crisis, such as an impending war, these women would be consulted by the political leaders (perhaps they would also *be* the political leaders) and they would go into meditation (for those still menstruating, during their moon-time). The knowledge of what action should or should not be taken would naturally emerge from them and would then be given to the larger community as a recommendation from the wise women of the land.

At the moment, many of our wise women are working in the background, exerting what influence they can on a world driven mad by materialism and lack of spiritual connection. It is time these women came to the foreground and changed the world. As Changing Woman herself spun the web of the beginning of time, so now she must emerge to shift the balance of power, so that the children of our children's children will have a world in which to live and love.

APPENDICES

Appendix i
Menstrual blood and blood-transmitted infections

Certain illnesses, most notably HIV, are transmitted through the blood. The HIV virus does not live for long outside the body because it needs the constant temperature of body heat to survive. This means that cloth pads soaked in cold water and then washed thoroughly in hot water are safe.

Where this issue can affect us is in the practice of ceremony involving menstrual blood as sacrament. As a general rule, if you are going to use blood ceremonially make sure that women only come into contact with their own blood. Unfortunately we can no longer share our body fluids with each other without great caution. Historically, the sharing of blood in ritual has been a major ingredient in bonding individuals and groups, but we live in a time where this is no longer safe.

Appendix ii
Update on cervical dysplasia

My upsetting visits with the gynecologist from patriarchal hell, described in Chapter Four, took place in the early 1980's. Much changed during the 1980's and 1990's and now there are many more women gynecologists, as well as a greater awareness among gynecologists of both genders about the respectful treatment of women. We still have a way to go, but my story should in no way deter women from seeking professional help if they have worrying menstrual or vaginal symptoms, or from having regular cervical screening.

More is known now about the nature of cervical dysplasia and the human papilloma virus (HPV), which appears to be a significant factor. I say "appears", because there are still conundrums which are not explained by the reductionist medical model; for example, one study found that HPV was detected in the cells of around 50% of the people studied, yet a much smaller percentage actually get genital warts, and an even smaller percentage of women go on to develop dysplasia, so there are clearly other factors at work. Warts have always been considered to be a mysterious malady, amenable to magical remedies and spells, and I am sure there is much we do not understand about the psychological element at play here.

Along with many other people, and supported by growing research evidence, I believe that contributory factors include the body's immune response which is now known to be directly affected by the individual's emotional state. One's emotional state is affected directly by one's self-love, or lack thereof. In both women and men, the reproductive organs are a prime area in which lack of self-love and self-acceptance is expressed somatically.

As well as understanding the causation of cervical dysplasia in greater depth, there are also new treatment modalities, surgical and non-surgical. The LEEP procedure is more specific than cauterization or cone biopsy, targeting the area of dysplasia rather than the whole cervix.

In recent years, naturopaths have been developing herbal treatments for dysplasia and achieving impressive results combining vitamin therapy with suppositories. There are some excellent products now available from naturopathic and herbal companies, specifically for the treatment of dysplasia. The relationship between dysplasia and menstrual disturbance is still not understood in Western medicine, or even recognized to exist.

NOTES

Preface
1. Research by Joanne Leslie, UCLA Dept. of Public Health and Pacific Women's Institute.

Chapter One
1. Marija Gimbutas, *The Language of the Goddess*; Merlin Stone, *When God Was a Woman*.
2. Although the Jewish religion had a long tradition of menstrual taboos (part of the Laws of Niddah), similar taboos were not common in European culture until the middle ages when Theodore, the author of an influential medieval penitential, stated that it was a sin for a menstruating woman to enter a church, and he imposed a penance for infraction of this rule. See G. Rattray Taylor, *Sex in History*, 59.
3. Dr. W. C. Taylor, *A Physician's Counsels to Women in Health and Disease* (1871), quoted in *Complaints and Disorders, The Sexual Politics of Sickness*, Ehrenreich and English, 21.
4. Dr. F. Hollick, *The Diseases of Women* (1849), quoted in Ehrenreich and English, 29.
5. Dr. W. W. Bliss, *Woman and her Thirty Years' Pilgrimage* (1870) quoted in Ehrenreich and English, 29.
6. Germaine Greer, *The Female Eunuch* (London: Paladin, 1971): 51-52.

Chapter Two
1. Elinor Gadon, *The Once & Future Goddess*, 2.
2. Barbara Walker, *The Woman's Encyclopedia of Myths and Secrets*, 669.
3. W. Carew Hazlitt, *Faiths and Folklores of the British Isles*, 418.
4. Wendy Doniger O'Flaherty, *Hindu Myths* (Harmondsworth: England, Penguin Books, 1975): 89.
5. C.G. Jung, *Man and His Symbols*, 276.
6. Claudia de Lys, *The Giant Book of Superstitions*, 414.
7. Lindsay River and Sally Gillespie, *The Knot of Time*, 69.
8. Despite this lack of religious female deities, it is interesting to observe the rise in prominence of secular goddesses in recent years, such as the late cultural icon Diana, Princess of Wales.

9.   Claudia de Lys, *The Giant Book of Superstitions*, 458.
10. Hazlitt, *Faiths and Folklores of the British Isles*, 417.
11. Buckley, "Menstruation and the Power of Yurok Women," in *Blood Magic*, ed. Thomas Buckley and Alma Gottlieb, 191.
12. Penelope Shuttle and Peter Redgrove, *The Wise Wound*, 284.
13. Gadon, *The Once & Future Goddess*, 6.
14. Walker, *The Woman's Encyclopedia of Myths and Secrets*, 635.
15. Ibid., 638.
16. Ibid., 638.
17. Ajit Mookerjee, *Kali. The Feminine Force*, 33.
18. Walker, *The Woman's Encyclopedia of Myths and Secrets*, 636-637.
19. Shuttle and Redgrove, *The Wise Wound*, 182.
20. Gadon, *The Once and Future Goddess*, 11.
21. The concept of sacrifice is complex and wide-ranging in human experience. Sacrifice is used in many societies as an attempt to ward off the harsh hand of fate by placating the gods in advance. This may be unconnected with ancient rituals involving menstrual blood.
22. Alan Ereira, *The Heart of the World*, BBC documentary, 1991.
23. Walker, *The Woman's Encyclopedia of Myths and Secrets*, 265.

Chapter Three

1.   Anne Cameron, *Daughters of Copper Woman*, 103.
2.   Ibid., 57.
3.   Buckley, "Menstruation and the Power of Yurok Women," in *Blood Magic*, 190.
4.   Cameron, *Daughters of Copper Woman*, 102-3.
5.   Ibid., 102.
6.   Colin Turnbull, *The Forest People*, 187.
7.   Ibid, 194.
8.   Sobonfu Somé, *The Spirit of Intimacy*, 71.
9.   Ibid., 73.
10. Ibid., 73.
11. Turnbull, 93. (italics mine)

Chapter Four

1.   Cervical dysplasia can be a precursor to cervical cancer. It is most important to have regular check-ups if you are diagnosed with dysplasia, and your doctor will advise you if treatment is necessary.

Chapter Five

1. Austen, *Heart of the Goddess*, 116.
2. Frazer, *The Golden Bough*, 700.
3. Claudia de Lys, *The Giant Book of Superstitions*, 46.
4. Frazer, *The Golden Bough*, 795.
5. Denise L. Lawrence, "Menstrual Politics: Women and Pigs in Rural Portugal," in *Blood Magic*, ed. Buckley and Gottlieb, 122.
6. Arnold Mindell, *The Dreambody in Relationships* (London: Routledge & Kegan, Paul, 1985).
7. Personal communication, Sebastopol, CA, Dec. 1990.
8. Susan M. Lark M.D., *PMS: A Self-Help Guide for Women* (update 1990).
9. Ibid., 2.
10. Ibid., 2.
11. Arnold Mindell, *Working with the Dreaming Body* (London: Routledge & Kegan, Paul, 1985).
12. See *The Wild Genie* by Alexandra Pope in which she tellls her story of learning to process severe menstrual pain.
13. A study of the menstrual behavior of 53 American women found that: "Nearly everyone listed a quiet relaxing activity as what they like to do during menstruation e.g. read, stay in bed, be alone, sleep, paint, write, garden, take it easy, meditate, take baths." Taylor, *Red Flower: Rethinking Menstruation*, 112.

Chapter Six

1. M. Esther Harding, *Women's Mysteries, Ancient and Modern* (Boston: Shambhala, 1990): 62-63.
2. Robert Briffault, *The Mothers*, abridged by Gordon Rattray Taylor (New York: Atheneum, 1977): 253.
3. Walker, *The Woman's Encyclopedia of Myths and Secrets*, 1020.
4. Monica Sjoo and Barbara Mor, *The Great Cosmic Mother*, Harper & Row, 189.
5. Ann Belford Ulanov, *The Feminine in Jungian Psychology and in Christian Theology* (Evanston IL.: Northwestern University Press, 1971): 176.
6. Mookerjee, *Kali: The Feminine Force*, 32-35.

Chapter Eight

1. Connie Kaplan, Dream Class, Santa Monica, CA, 7/31/96.
2. Patricia Garfield, *Women's Bodies, Women's Dreams* (New York:

Ballantine, 1988): 74 – 79.

3. Gary Dale Richman, "The Santo Daime Doctrine", in *Shaman's Drum* 22 (Winter 1990-91): 35.

Chapter Thirteen
1. Interview with Susun Weed by Marcelina Martin, 1990.
2. Sobonfu Somé, *The Spirit of Intimacy*, 74.
3. Steve Deese and Debbie Heartsong, personal correspondence, 1991.

Chapter Fourteen
1. Hallie Iglehart Austin, *The Heart of the Goddess.*
2. Chris Knight, *Blood Relations: Menstruation and the Origins of Culture,* 36.
3. H. H. the 14th Dalai Lama, public address on world peace, Los Angeles, June 6 1997.

Selected Bibliography

Anthropology

Beck, Peggy and Anna Walters. *The Sacred: Ways of Knowledge, Sources of Life*. Tsaile, AZ: Navajo Community College Press, 1977.

Briffault, Robert. *The Mothers*. Abridged by G. Rattray Taylor. New York: Atheneum, 1977.

Buckley, Thomas & Alma Gottlieb, eds. *Blood Magic: The Anthropology of Menstruation*. Berkeley and Los Angeles: University of California, 1988.

Cameron, Anne. *Daughters of Copper Woman*. Vancouver: Press Gang, 1981.

Eliade, Mircea. *Rites and Symbols of Initiation*. New York: Harper & Row, 1958.

Ereira, Alan. *The Heart of the World*. London: Jonathan Cape, 1990.

Knight, Chris. *Blood Relations: Menstruation and the Origins of Culture*. New Haven, CT: Yale University Press, 1991.

Lawlor, Robert. *Voices of the First Day: Awakening in the Aboriginal Dreamtime*. Rochester, VT: Inner Traditions International, 1991.

Mahdi, Louise, Steven Foster and Meredith Little, eds. *Betwixt & Between*. La Salle, IL: Open Court, 1987.

Shostak, Marjorie. *Nisa: The Life and Words of a Kung Woman*. New York: Vintage, 1981.

Somé, Sobonfu E. *The Spirit of Intimacy*. Berkeley: Berkeley Hill Books, 1997.

Turnbull, Colin. *The Forest People*. New York: Simon & Schuster, 1961.

Goddess Studies

Austen, Hallie Iglehart. *The Heart of the Goddess*. Berkeley, CA: Wingbow, 1990.

Eisler, Riane. *The Chalice and the Blade*. San Francisco: Harper & Row, 1987.

Gadon, Elinor. *The Once & Future Goddess*. San Francisco: Harper & Row, 1989.

Getty, Adele. *Goddess: Mother of Living Nature*. New York: Thames & Hudson, 1990.

Gimbutas, Marija. *The Language of the Goddess*. San Francisco: Harper & Row, 1989.

Mookerjee, Ajit. *Kali, The Feminine Force*. Rochester, VT: Destiny Books, 1988.

Noble, Vicki. *Motherpeace: A Way to the Goddess through Myth, Art, and Tarot*. San Francisco: Harper & Row, 1983.

Noble, Vicki. *Shakti Woman*. San Francisco: HarperSanFrancisco, 1991.

Sjoo, Monica, and Barbara Mor. *The Great Cosmic Mother*. San Francisco: Harper & Row, 1987.

Stone, Merlin. *When God was a Woman*. New York: Harvest/Harcourt Brace Jovanovich, 1976.

Menstruation

Francia, Luisa. *Dragontime*. Woodstock: Ash Tree Publishing, 1988.

Golub, Sharon. *Periods: From Menarche to Menopause*. Newbury Park, CA: Sage Publications, 1992.

Lark, Susan M., M.D. *PMS: Premenstrual Syndrome, Self Help Book*. Berkeley, CA: Celestial Arts 1984.

Shuttle, Penelope, and Peter Redgrove. *The Wise Wound.* New York: Grove Press 1978, 1986.

Taylor, Dena. *Red Flower: Rethinking Menstruation.* Freedom, CA: The Crossing Press, 1988.

Mythology

de Lys, Claudia. *The Giant Book of Superstitions.* Secaucus, N.J.: Citadel Press, 1979.

Frazer, J. G. *The Golden Bough: A Study in Magic and Religion.* New York: Macmillan, 1922.

Hazlitt, W. Carew. *Faiths and Folklores of the British Isles.* (2 vols) New York: Benjamin Bloom, 1965.

Jung, C. G. *Man and His Symbols.* New York: Dell, 1968.

Knight, Richard Payne. *The Symbolical Language of Ancient Art & Mythology.* New York: J. W. Bouton, 1892.

Graves, Robert. *The Greek Myths.* New York: Penguin, 1955.

Walker, Barbara. *The Woman's Encyclopedia of Myths & Secrets.* San Francisco: Harper & Row, 1983.

Natural Medicine

Crawford, Amanda McQuade. *The Herbal Menopause Book* (contains recipes and advice for perimenopausal women and menstrual problems), Freedom, CA: The Crossing Press, 1996.

Gladstar, Rosemary. *Herbal Healing for Women.* New York: Fireside 1993.

McIntyre, Anne. *Complete Woman's Herbal.* Henry Holt 1994.

Northrup, Dr. Christiane. *Women's Bodies, Women's Wisdom.* New York: Bantam, 1994.

Tisserand, Robert. *The Art of Aromatherapy*. New York: Inner Traditions International, 1977.

Weed, Susan. *Healing Wise*. Woodstock, NY: Ash Tree Publishing, 1989.

Psychology

Mindell, Arnold. *Working with the Dreaming Body*. London: Routledge & Kegan Paul, 1985.

Mindell, Arnold. *Working on Yourself Alone*. London: Arkana, 1990.

Women's Studies

Ehrenreich, Barbara, and Deirdre English. *Complaints and Disorders: The Sexual Politics of Sickness*. New York: The Feminist Press, 1973.

Garfield, Patricia. *Women's Bodies, Women's Dreams*. New York: Ballantine, 1988.

Martin, Emily. *The Woman in the Body: A Cultural Analysis of Reproduction*. New York: Beacon Press, 1987.

Hall, Nor. *The Moon and the Virgin*. New York: Harper & Row, 1980.

Harding, M. Esther. *Women's Mysteries, Ancient and Modern*. Boston: Shambhala, 1990.

River, Lindsay, and Sally Gillespie. *The Knot of Time: Astrology and the Female Experience*. New York: Harper & Row, 1987.

Rush, Anne Kent. *Moon, Moon*. New York: Random House, 1976.

Spretnak, Charlene, ed. *The Politics of Women's Spirituality*. New York: Doubleday, 1982.

Zweig, Connie, ed. *To Be a Woman: The Birth of the Conscious Feminine*. Los Angeles: Jeremy Tarcher, 1990.

ABOUT THE AUTHOR

Lara Owen was born in England in 1955. She was educated at Nottingham High School for Girls and graduated from the University of Warwick. She then studied Chinese medicine in England and China, and established one of the first multidisciplinary holistic health centers in the UK.

After practicing as a doctor of Chinese medicine for most of the 1980's, Lara moved to California and began to write. *Her Blood Is Gold* was her first book and was inspired and informed by her experiences on retreat in wilderness areas, and from spiritual practice and study in the Native American and Tibetan Buddhist traditions.

Lara now lives in southwest England. For information about her books, her teaching schedule, and her work with individuals and groups, please visit http://laraowen.com.

OTHER TITLES BY ARCHIVE PUBLISHING

for full details please see our website

www.archivepublishing.co.uk
and
transpersonalbooks.com

The Dark Moon *Anne Maria Clarke*
A Twist in Coyote's Tale *Celia M Gunn*
Performing the Dreams of your Body *Dr. Jill Hayes*

and in the wisdom of the transpersonal series written by
Ian Gordon-Brown and *Barbara Somers*
Series Editor *Hazel Marshall*

Journey in Depth: A Transpersonal Perspective
The Fires of Alchemy: A Transpersonal Viewpoint
The Raincloud of Knowable Things:
A Practical Guide to Transpersonal Psychology

other titles distributed by Archive and written by
Bryce Taylor
Working with Others
Forging the Future Together
Learning for Tomorrow: Wholeperson Learning